MUSCLE

CONFESSIONS
OF AN
UNLIKELY
BODYBUILDER

SAMUEL WILSON FUSSELL

AVON BOOKS ◆ NEW YORK

AVON BOOKS
A division of
The Hearst Corporation
1350 Avenue of the Americas
New York, New York 10019

Copyright © 1991 by Samuel Wilson Fussell
Cover art by Larry Ratzkin
Cover photograph by John R. Coletti copyright © 1991
Published by arrangement with Poseidon Press, Simon and Schuster, Inc.
Library of Congress Catalog Card Number: 90-47085
ISBN: 0-380-71763-8

The Poseidon Press edition contains the following Library of Congress Cataloging in Publication data:

Fussell, Samuel Wilson.
  Muscle: confessions of an unlikely bodybuilder / Samuel Wilson Fussell.
      p. cm.
  1. Fussell, Samuel Wilson. 2. Bodybuilders—United States—Biography. I. Title.
GV545.52.F87A3   1991
646.7'5—dc20
[B]   90-47085
                                         CIP

First Avon Books Trade Printing: August 1992

AVON TRADEMARK REG. U.S. PAT. OFF. AND IN OTHER COUNTRIES, MARCA REGISTRADA, HECHO EN U.S.A.

Printed in the U.S.A.

OPM 10 9 8 7 6 5 4

MUSCLE

To Peter Conrad

ALTHOUGH THE FOLLOWING ACCOUNT IS TRUE, THE NAMES OF CERTAIN PERSONS AND PLACES HAVE BEEN CHANGED IN THE INTEREST OF PRESERVING THEIR ANONYMITY AND PROTECTING MY OWN LIFE.

S.W.F.

CONTENTS

WHEN YOU OPERATE IN AN OVERBUILT ME-
TROPOLIS, YOU HAVE TO HACK YOUR WAY
WITH A MEAT AX.

—ROBERT MOSES

THE FIRST DUTY IN LIFE IS TO ASSUME A POSE.
WHAT THE SECOND IS, NO ONE HAS YET DIS-
COVERED.

—OSCAR WILDE

THE INTRODUCTION

You spot them on the streets of the city and, increasingly, in the malls and parks of the suburbs. Sometimes they band together. Mostly, they walk alone. Bodybuilders. You know the kind. They strut like no others, holding their elbows wider than their shoulders, legs far apart. I know, I was one of them.

For four long years, I trained four hours a day, six days a week with them. I broke whole wheat bread with them. I filled my body with steroids alongside them. I lived with them. And, finally, I competed on stage against them.

The following is an account of my journey—what I did, what I saw, what I felt. Those in search of a steroid primer or an exercise manual are advised to look elsewhere; my purpose is different. Part ditty, part dirge, I sing of arms and the man, of weight rooms and muscle pits, of biceps and triceps, bench presses and low pulley rows, of young and old, woman and man, straining and hoisting iron to the boom box sound of Top 40 record stations in bodybuilding gyms across the land.

I sing of dreamers and addicts, rogues and visionaries. And I sing of my own solitary pilgrimage into this strange world. A world filled with wrist straps and ammonia, BIG Chewables and "the juice." A world governed by a savage force that swallowed me whole from a bookstore in New York City, and did not relent until it had chewed me up and spit me out 80 pounds heavier and 3,000 miles later on a posing dais in Burbank, California. I was swabbed in posing oil and competition color, flexing with all my might, when I came to, a sadder and wiser man.

1.

THE GENESIS

ALL THE UNHAPPINESS OF MAN STEMS FROM
ONE THING ONLY: THAT HE IS INCAPABLE OF
STAYING QUIETLY IN HIS ROOM.

—PASCAL

Bodybuilders call it "the disease." Its symptoms include a complete commitment to all matters pertaining to iron. Not the kind of iron you use to press your clothes, but the kind they use to create bulges and muscular mounds in their bodies. You find "the diseased" in bookstores hovering by the rack containing the muscle magazines (invariably adjacent to the pornography). You overhear them in vitamin stores, discussing the merits of branch-chain amino acids and protein powders. You scan them on the subway, their hypertrophied bodies a silent, raging scream of dissent. And, walking to work in the morning, you can see them through the windows of their gyms, hoisting and heaving weights in a lifting frenzy.

Most of them catch the disease during the years of adolescence. On the back pages of comic books, scrawny teens find advertisements for chest expanders and chin-up bars. For many that's where the affair ends: in an unmailed letter or as cobwebbed, unused equipment piled in the basement. But for a few—the truly afflicted— the arrival of the equipment is just the beginning. Within a matter of months, they graduate from chest expanders to bench presses, from pull-ups to squats. Eventually, as their bodies fill out and the dream takes hold, they gravitate from distant neighborhoods to their own kind in the gyms of the city.

This was not my story. I passed into my mid-twenties knowing nothing of the disease. Until the age of twenty-six, in fact, my life was filled with books. I began my course of reading at a prep school called Lawrenceville and continued it through my graduation from Oxford University. Until then, everything was set. The son of two university professors of English, I was next in line to assume the academic mantle. My parents' only cause for concern was the fact that I preferred American literature to English.

The trouble began when I moved back to New York City for a year off after Oxford before I was to enter graduate school. Within a month I found a sublet on the Upper East Side and a job in publishing. But suddenly and spectacularly my health began to deteriorate. First it was my lungs (the doctors diagnosed pleurisy), then it was a fever (this time, pneumonia). Despite medications, my condition did not improve. Colds, hot flashes, chills—one malady replaced another.

My arrival at work every morning set off a communal buzz of concern. At six feet four and 170 pounds sopping wet, I had always been gaunt. But now, with rasping lungs and cadaverous complexion, I looked like an outpatient from Bellevue (which, in fact, I was). I publicly tried to pass off my predicament as nothing serious—I was just feeling a little under the weather, I said. Things would take a turn for the better come spring, I was sure of it.

And my friends averred that this must be the case. They took me out to lunch and tried to take my mind off my health. But all along, I knew the cause of my own particular disorder; I was just loath to admit it. The problem, you see, was New York. It terrified me. To divulge my fears seemed cowardly, somehow unworthy of the city. But finally, among the lunch gathering, bracketed by a coughing fit, I let it all out. Was I the only one, I asked haltingly, living in a constant state of terror in the city? Did others also find themselves under siege?

As soon as I admitted it, the facts and figures came tumbling out of my mouth. The rapes, the muggings, the assaults, the murders. Those were the majors, but the minors were just as bad. I felt trapped by the teeming populace, dwarfed by skyscrapers, suffocated by the fumes from factories and expressways. And then there was Jerry, and men like him.

"Jerry?" they asked.

I was surprised they didn't know him. He seemed to be on a first name basis with much of the city.

"Hi, Jews for Jesus! Jerry here—that's with a J!" he would shout, as soon as he spotted my head on the subway escalator each morning at Grand Central. Sandwich board and all, he waited for me at the top of the platform, plucking *me* out from the hundreds of other commuters fore and aft.

"How ya doin, Stretch?" he'd begin, all smiles and concern, draping an arm around my shoulder. And then, in an abrupt change of tone, he'd pounce: "What I mean to say is . . . how do you feel about . . . *tomorrow?*"

I explained to growing laughter around the table that Jerry was just one of many "friends" drawn to me through the course of the day like slivers of steel to a magnet. Something about me seemed to appeal to every deadbeat, con artist, and self-proclaimed philosopher of the city. No matter where I turned, confidence tricksters hounded my path.

At the conclusion of my painful monologue, I sat back exhausted, shamed that I was so vulnerable. And then, suddenly, merry voices chimed in from all sides at the table. Apparently, I'd struck a chord after all. There was Niels, who exulted in the fact that his wet, limp clothes had been scattered across the laundromat floor by a street tough when he hadn't removed them from the washer on time. There was Matthew, rocking in his chair in delight, as he told us of the gray-suited man who followed him home one day, lowered his trousers on Matthew's doorstep in mid-afternoon, and defecated on his welcome mat. Troopers together, everyone seemed to have their stories to tell.

What had happened in the recent past to the newscaster Dan Rather had, in one form or another, happened to us all. Two men had accosted Rather on the street, and took turns beating him, all the while asking him the question: "What is the frequency, Kenneth?" Self-consciously, I joined the laughter at the table in the retelling of the story. It was agreed that the fact that it made no sense made perfect sense.

"Urban dissonance," my friends called it, the inevitable result of the great flux of cultures and tribes, languages and races that make up the city. Too many people, too little space. The result: noise, stench, subway riders pushed in front of trains—all unavoidable by-products of "modernism."

Urban dissonance was one thing—diarrhea another. The city

literally scared the shit out of me. It wasn't just Jerry or the crowds, the heckling or the hassles. It wasn't just bag ladies lamenting their persecution by the CIA. It wasn't even the nightly serenade of gunshots and sirens outside my bedroom window. These things I might someday learn to cope with. Try as I might, there were things I simply couldn't ignore.

Like what I'd witnessed on a downtown subway platform my first month back in the city. All I could hear at first were the screams, but as I neared I saw the crowd. They were milling around two men, one a huge, bearded skell (a man who lives in the tunnels and trains beneath the city) and in his grasp, a hapless businessman. The skell was shaking him like a rag doll while the victim shrieked in fear. No one made a move to help him. We all watched, paralyzed, as the skell punched his victim repeatedly in the face. Every blow he struck sounded like a baseball bat hitting a side of ham. It was beyond brutal, and when the skell grew bored at last and skipped away, leaving his prey comatose in a pool of blood, we heard him far down the subway corridor singing a nursery rhyme in victory.

I realized the god-awful truth when I helped the poor man to his feet. It could just as easily have been me, just as I could have been the one strolling down First Avenue at the precise moment an air conditioner dropped from a fourth story window. As it was, according to the papers, it was one Elizabeth Beaugrand who was brained. Just a matter of time before it would be my turn, and if it wasn't an air conditioner, then it might well be a construction crane, a snapping bridge cable, a cement block, or, of course, a knife, fist, gun, or rug cutter.

My New York days I spent running wide-eyed in fear down city streets, my nights passed in closeted toilet-bound terror in my sublet. My door triple-locked, windows nailed shut, the curtains, needless to say, drawn. The place was going to explode at any moment—I could feel it—and unless I gained something fast, some uniform, some velcro, I would catapult into oblivion along with the rest of the shards. Caught in this nightmare, I needed something, anything, to secure my safety.

My friends advised me to try the usual anodynes: Something like The Harvard Club or The New York Society Library might do the trick. A lit candle in a dark room. And if not that, well then, why not some exercise, like Tae Kwon Do even, or, if need be, Plato's Retreat? In any case, don't worry, they said. Just stop taking things so seriously.

But how could I stop taking things so seriously when conditions were so serious? A recent MIT study indicated that a combat soldier had had a better chance surviving World War II than a New Yorker surviving New York.

My family was out. I couldn't retreat to our house in Princeton because it had been sold while I was away at Oxford. After thirty years of marriage, my parents had bitterly and publicly divorced. To choose one parent's home would have meant taking sides. I did try a girlfriend, and we spent a number of blissful afternoons together. But the partings were always hell. She had to rush off each evening to the downtown apartment she shared with her fiancé.

The more I learned about the city, the more I noticed the alternatives. Suicide, for one.

BOY GULPS
GAS, EXPLODES!

So the New York *Post* reported. On an average of once a week, a citizen leaps to the tracks in a subway station to kiss the third rail or jumps to his death in front of an oncoming train. The George Washington Bridge is another favored spot, along with the few skyscrapers still lacking the deterrent of fences and barbed wire on their peaks.

Finding an activity was another alternative. In Washington Square Park on weekends I found scores of men, heads burrowed in their hands, playing chess, all in quest of regulation and safety in the square grid of the chessboard. I saw white men dressed in black on the subway, swaying in their seats, reciting Talmudic texts aloud. I saw black men dressed in white, periodically unfurling prayer rugs and chanting toward Islam.

Relocation was another possible solution: heading off in a silver camper with an untainted water supply to the mountain peaks of the West, proclaiming myself a "survivalist." (I'd noticed that survivalists of a different stripe relocated to places like Taos, New

Mexico, and called themselves "artists.") But I didn't want to relocate. I just wanted to be less assailable, less vulnerable. Good God, it was enough to make a grown man cry, or—hold your hats—turn to bodybuilding.

I was ducking for cover, as usual, when it happened. This time it was a man with a crowbar and a taxi medallion, worth $50,000 at the going rate, which he had just ripped off the hood of a New York taxi cab. Spotting me as a likely customer, he'd advanced upon me, brandishing the crowbar for emphasis. I quickly sought shelter in the nearest building, which turned out to be the New York landmark, The Strand bookstore. It was an appropriate refuge—I'd used books all my life for protection. I caught my breath and, as was my custom, made way to the autobiography section (I frequently found myself there wondering how *they* coped with life).

It was in this aisle, in this store, in September of 1984, that I finally caught "the disease." Here it was I came across *Arnold: The Education of a Bodybuilder* by Arnold Schwarzenegger. A glimpse of the cover told me all I needed to know. There he stood on a mountain top in Southern California, every muscle bulging to the world as he flexed and smiled and posed. Just the expression on his face indicated that nothing could disturb this man. A victim? Not bloody likely.

As for his body, why, here was protection, and loads of it. What were these great chunks of tanned, taut muscle but modern-day armor? Here were breastplates, greaves, and pauldrons aplenty, and all made from human flesh. He had taken stock of his own situation and used the weight room as his smithy. A human fortress—a perfect defense to keep the enemy host at bay. What fool would dare storm those foundations?

And that's where it hit me, right there in The Strand. I knew it in an instant, my prayers were answered. What if I made myself a walking billboard of invulnerability like Arnold? Why couldn't *I* use muscles as insurance, as certain indemnity amidst the uncertainty of urban strife? Arnold had used iron to his obvious advantage, why couldn't I? And if the price was high, as a quick glance at the tortured faces in the training photos suggested, well, wouldn't four hours a day of private pain be worth a lifetime of public safety?

Nothing else had worked for me. The Harvard Club tie and The New York Society Library card had done nothing to ward off attack. As for Tae Kwon Do, one had to actually engage in street combat to use it. But muscles—big, loud muscles—well, they were something else altogether. Surely a quick appraisal of my new gargantuan body would guarantee me immunity, even from the criminally insane. And the beauty of it all lay in the probable fact that I would never be called upon actually to *use* these muscles. I could remain a coward and no one would ever know!

It was that simple at first—at least, so I thought. By making myself larger than life, I might make myself a little less frail, a little less assailable when it came down to it, a little less human. In the beginning I planned to use bodybuilding purely as a system of self-defense. It wasn't until later, 80 muscle-crammed pounds later, that I learned to use it as my principal method of assault.

2.

THE Y

WE ARE ALL STILL PIONEERS, REQUIRED TO COLONIZE THE PIECE OF GROUND WHICH CHANCE ASSIGNS US, TO MAKE IT OUR OWN BY SHAPING IT INTO A SMALL, AUTONOMOUS, INTELLIGIBLE WORLD.

—PETER CONRAD

I spent the next day at work educating myself about the lifting world. I wanted to make sure that I entered the gym that night with the appropriate attitude. The preparation, I felt, was essential—the sooner I built myself up, the sooner I'd find safety. So it was that I spent that morning ignoring my typing chores and underlining passages from *Arnold: The Education of a Bodybuilder.* By noon, I'd practically memorized the whole text.

I was too nervous to eat at lunch, and found myself instead in a magazine store, shelling out money for muscle periodicals. *Flex, Power, Ironman, Muscular Development, Muscle & Fitness*—I got them all, and passed the afternoon in my cubicle going through the glossy pages.

I skimmed over the photos showing the models with their gaunt cheeks and wasted, scrawny frames. From the beginning, I never had the slightest interest in what the magazines called "toning" or "spot reduction." These models reminded me of myself as I was, not as I wanted to be. How would a low percentage of body fat help me in the event of a street fracas?

I wanted to get as big as possible as fast as possible. The bigger, the better—that boded best for personal protection. So it was the most massive bodybuilders who caught my eye. Builders whose flexed arms were actually larger than their heads. Builders who could balance a glass of milk on top of their inflated chests. Builders like the Cuban expatriate Sergio Oliva (now a cop in Chicago), Bertil ("Beef It") Fox, Geoff ("Neck") King.

These men never sucked in their cheeks. Just the opposite, they puffed and preened through the pages, displaying their frightening wares of tanned tissue and bulging veins in the most Herculean poses: the crab, the javelin throw, the back double-biceps. And always, every few pages, there was Arnold.

The Education had been clear on Arnold's history. Born in 1948 to middle-class parents in Graz, Austria, he began his communion with iron at the age of fifteen. He approached the weights with what Gaines and Butler in their book *Pumping Iron* labeled such "joy and fierceness" that just five years later, barely out of his teens, he won his first Mr. Universe title. By the time he retired, "The Austrian Oak" had won Mr. Universe four more times and the most prestigious title in bodybuilding, Mr. Olympia, an unprecedented seven times. Arnold ruled bodybuilding in the way Muhammad Ali ruled boxing, with enough skill and charisma to dumbfound critics and competitors alike.

But it didn't end there. Upon his retirement from bodybuilding, Arnold simply changed fields, making himself part of the Zeitgeist with his ascension to the silver screen and his marriage to Maria Shriver.

Through iron, he had got what he wanted: big-balled muscles and a permanent pass to the Kennedy compound. Surely, I thought at my desk, if he could do that, then I could fulfill my own more limited ambition and gain 20 to 30 pounds.

But I had a feeling it wouldn't be easy. Gone were the days of Indian clubs and Charles Atlas. I had seen a photo of him once, smiling and flexing on the beach, supporting a pair of bathing beauties on his broad shoulders. He made lifting seem as easy and pleasant as a Sunday afternoon stroll in the park.

In the pages of the magazines spread out before me, however, there was not a smile to be found on these modern-day builders. Just a look of grim determination, as lifter after lifter grunted, strained, heaved, and pulled black iron in California gyms. They seemed close to bursting from the stress. How far they'd come from the days of Charles Atlas. It was not at all clear that these modern men were even of the same species.

I sat in my cubicle and inhaled anxiously. I hadn't counted on the pain angle—not to this degree anyway. I wavered just for a moment, but then made my decision. If this "no pain, no gain" adage were true, then, I would learn not just to accept pain, but to embrace it.

With that resolve, I found myself after work grimly purchasing the necessities for my mission. I bought a stiff leather weight-lifting belt, a pair of canvas sneakers, jocks, and gray sweats. What else would I need? Bandages? A stretcher? Clutching my new gym bag to my bony chest, I made it to the Vanderbilt Y on East Forty-seventh Street, just a few blocks from my job. With my corporate discount, the price was negligible.

There I sat in my black, size 38-L suit, as Mr. Quigley, the head membership coordinator, spoke to me of the advantages of the gym.

"We've got jogging," he said, "though, of course, you have to run in packs. . . ."

"Packs?" I asked, confused.

"Yes," he sighed. "For safety's sake. To lessen the probability factor of attack by EDPs on the street."

"EDPs?" I asked.

"Yes, you know, Emotionally Disturbed People."

I knew. The subway skell and his ilk—the reason I was there. I barely heard Mr. Quigley as he ran through the Y's other sports programs: basketball, swimming, karate. I didn't hear him at all when he spoke of ceramics, modern dance, and acting. I couldn't, the din upstairs was deafening. Mr. Quigley lifted his head and frowned as the ceiling quaked and white specks of plaster rained down on our heads.

"The weight room?" I asked, unable to contain my excitement.

"It makes me physically ill," Mr. Quigley grimaced. He shook his head sadly. The sagging heavy jowels, the eyes ringed with fatigue made him look like a rheumy basset hound. "Perverts. Animals. We don't like these people any more than you do," he said. "We don't encourage them, you understand, but we can't just stop them from coming in. We are, after all, a *Christian* organization."

This struck me as odd. After all, just that afternoon *The Education* had cleared up my own misconceptions. Arnold had stated categorically that the weight room was *not* a breeding ground for cripples and addicts, sexual deviants and dangerously unbalanced men. No, that was a false and absurd surmise from a prejudiced public, he'd said.

The muscle magazines concurred, taking great pains to explain that gyms are actually a haven of safety in a world rife with disease, poverty, and prejudice. They are the stronghold of democracy, they said, where every lifter, regardless of color or creed, is free to pursue personal physique gains. Just bring a "positive mental attitude," and you'll be among like-minded friends in the gym, the magazines promised, happy, healthy, and feeling terrific.

So, in some confusion, I pocketed the new membership card Mr. Quigley gave me, and headed up the steps to the Y's locker room that night. I pulled my new sweatshirt over my head, and collected myself on the wooden bench by my locker before venturing to the weight room.

"Remember," I prodded myself, hitting my fist into my cupped hand, "joy and fierceness," "joy and fierceness." I leaped up and strode to the door. It wasn't until I actually set a foot inside that I panicked.

First, it was the heat. It felt like a Saigon summer. My legs buckled from it. Then the crowd—I was amazed the room could hold them all. Everywhere around me, there were men. Hundreds of them. I say men, mind you, because, despite what the magazines suggested ("Lifting is *family fun!*"), there were no women or children present.

I recognized the fierceness immediately. The air was filled with violence. On the far side of the room, among the scattered dumbbells and barbells—the "free-weights" I recognized from the magazines—gathered a muscular band of men about ten strong. Many of them wore camouflage pants and black combat boots. They punctuated their exercises with savage screams and directed murderous glances toward the fifty or so thinner men who were working out near me.

The men on my side of the room were engaged in pulling cables or lifting bars connected to two skeletal, chrome structures immediately before me. All I could hear, aside from the background rock music, were wrenching groans of despair and the monotonous clinking of iron. All I could see beneath the sickly glow of the few working fluorescent bulbs were the sagging shoulders and bent brows of the defeated. So much for joy.

The floor was a dumbbell graveyard. A few were chrome, but most were flat, ugly, black iron, and they covered the interconnecting rubber black mats that passed for a rug. The walls, coated in dimpled black rubber, supported steel racks of all sizes, some apparently to accommodate certain exercises, others to house the iron equipment. The windows were covered with corroded iron bars. The whole hopeless thing looked like a nightmare out of Piranesi.

I hadn't the faintest idea how to proceed. Should I simply select one of the weights at my feet and start swinging it, as if I were an iron veteran? I bent forward to pick one of the smaller ones up from the floor, when a fist hit my kidney, and a scream pierced my ear.

"Move your ass, stork!"

I sagged to my knees from the blow and looked directly into the eyes of a double amputee. On his chest he wore a shirt that said Bert, on his head a baseball cap that said "Do the Hustle." He covered what was left of his legs with a Hefty garbage bag, drawn tight around his waist by his weight-lifting belt. There was no wheelchair in sight. The size of his massive arms made me wonder if he'd ever used one.

"I beg your pardon," I muttered, feeling my aching kidney with one hand, shamed that I had inconvenienced him. "Can I help you get a weight?" I asked, in an attempt to remedy the situation.

"Fuck off, new meat!" he roared, scuttling off to join his huge friends at the free-weight sector.

By the time I regained my feet, this raucous band turned on me. At first, the chant was barely audible above the thunderous pulse of rock music, but it soon grew deafening.

"New meat! New meat!" the group sang, led by Bert, the snarling gargoyle. "NEW MEAT! NEW MEAT!"

My heart started racing. I began to hyperventilate. This was something I hadn't encountered in *The Education* or the magazines. What's next? I wondered. Rape? Public hanging? I was preparing to

flee and abandon the whole endeavor for one of the Y's safer offerings—ceramics perhaps—when a figure sprang up from behind
the neighboring machine and grabbed my hand.

"Hi, I'm Austin and a Capricorn!" he shouted above the clamor
with a smile. Though he was a bag of bones himself, his T-shirt
read, "If you're going to be a bear, be a grizzly!"

I was too frightened to say a word. It might be a trap, I remember
thinking. Warily, I accepted his hand.

"Oh, don't worry about *those* sillies." He waved at the beefy troop
on the far side of the room. No longer chanting, they now bickered
among themselves and directed their fury at the Olympic barbells
and dumbbells in their hands.

"They don't mean any harm—not really," Austin assured me. "I
couldn't help but notice you before back in the banana republic,"
he tittered, motioning to the locker room.

I explained to Austin as politely as possible that I had come to
the Y with one intention only, and that was physical development.
He understood immediately.

"Jesus, what wouldn't we all give for a few more inches," he
sighed.

"Should I start with free-weights?" I asked.

"Sorry, babe," he said, putting his arm around my shoulder, "but
you've got to learn to walk before you can run."

He steered me away from the free-weight side, toward his
friends.

With Austin's help, I made the acquaintance of the two machines
that dominated this part of the room. These were called "the Uni-
versals," named after their manufacturer, The Universal Machine
Corporation based in Cedar Rapids, Iowa. They looked like the
kind of stripped-down equipment U.S. astronauts had left on the
moon. According to Austin, they would be my principal means of
physical transformation.

"What we're all doing here is called 'circuit training,' " Austin
said, grandly waving his arms at the men before us.

I looked at the men by the machines. Heads bowed, they trudged
from one exercise station to wait in line by another. They looked
about as happy as war-torn collaborators awaiting execution. The

only sound I heard from them was a mechanical recitation as they counted their repetitions during each set.

"It's called a 'circuit,' " said Austin. "As you can see, we all do a little tour around the machine, stopping at certain stations along the way. Doesn't matter which of the two machines you choose, they're duplicates to ease the congestion. Now, see, all you have to do is lie on a bench, sit on a stool, or stand, depending on the exercise, and push or pull a bar or cable connected to a weight stack in the machine. One complete tour of all the stations, about ten in all, is a circuit. That should take you about 30 minutes. Three complete circuits is a workout."

I peered into the machine's metal innards. There were numerous weight stacks within the rectangular frame of the contraption. Each stack was attached to a pulley or a bar projected outward to a stool or station.

"Is it safe?" I asked, prodding the cold steel of a weight stack with my finger.

Austin laughed at my anxiety. "Look, you're a Virgo, am I right or am I right? I *knew* it! You Virgos are so fussy. These machines are much safer than those free-weights over there, believe me."

I looked over at the free-weight section. Just then, a short black man with absurdly huge legs wrapped his fingers tightly around another man's neck.

"Sweepea, Goddamnit! Call me by my fuckin' name. I ain't Mousie! I'm The Portuguese Rambo, you fuck!" he screamed.

Sweepea's face was rapidly turning purple. I looked around the room. No one was even watching. I glanced back at Austin.

"Oh, it doesn't mean a thing. Mousie, oh, I mean 'The Portuguese Rambo'—he likes to be called that, you know—well, he's very excitable. This sort of thing happens every night. It's part of the process," Austin explained.

He brought my attention back to the machines. With the Universal, he said, the weight is always connected to the machine. You never have to balance it, just push or pull. With free-weights, there is no intermediary between you and the weights. If you lose your grip with them, you might well crush your face.

"Machines are less efficient than free-weights if you really want size, since they do some of the work for you, but they're a great place to start," Austin told me. I understood. I needed a few months on training wheels before tackling the real stuff.

"Look, I'll take you through your first circuit, if you like," Austin said.

He ushered me off to a Naugahyde bench dripping with sweat. I lay flat down on it and watched as he inserted a metal pin in the weight stack by my head. The stack in the machine was connected to a bar that jutted out over my chest. Twelve times, I pushed the bar from my chest to arm's length. I started turning beetroot-red after the eighth rep. This was my introduction to the bench press.

"Breathe!" Austin shouted, hovering over me. "Like you're having a baby!"

At the shoulder, or deltoid, press, I perfected my breathing. I sat on a stool facing the Universal, grabbed the bar by my shoulders with both hands, and pushed it over my head. I exhaled when I pushed the bar up, and inhaled when I eased it down. At the seated rowing station, I sat on the floor, my feet braced against the machine, and made like a collegiate rower, substituting a handgrip, cable and weight stack for an oar. This was for my back or "lats," as Austin called them (the abbreviated form of latissimus dorsi).

I learned that my arms were really divided into two muscles: triceps, or the back of the arm, and biceps, the bulge at the top. Austin adjusted the stack as I worked my triceps by pushing down on a bar cabled to the top of one of the machine's stations. For my biceps, I fell in line with the others, waited my turn, then grabbed a handlebar at thigh height and curled it up to my chest.

That was it for my upper body. Push or pull and recover; fall in line for the next exercise; push or pull and recover. It was a continuing theme. Already, I could feel a nasty degree of pain.

Austin laughed. "Believe me, it's perfectly normal. You see, you tear the muscle each time you work out. That's why you wait 48 hours before working the same muscle again. If you don't, you just flog the thing to death, and it's of no use to anyone."

Legs were next, broken down into my "quads" or quadriceps, the front of the thighs; "hams" or hamstrings, the back of the thighs;

and calves. The Universal had special steel pedals for exercising the quads. I settled myself into the Naugahyde chair, braced my arms on the metal grips by my hips, and pushed, 12 times.

Austin went next, then led me to the line for the leg curl station, where I lay flat on my stomach on a bench, fit my legs under a padded bar, and, bending at the knee, brought the bar up with my heels to touch my hamstrings for 12 repetitions.

My first circuit was complete at the calf station, where I stood on a narrow plank of wood, and raised myself on tiptoe and back down again using only my calves. The exercise seemed absurdly simple until Austin added a padded yoke to my shoulders connecting me to a weight stack in the machine.

That was it, upper and lower body. I'd just completed my first circuit. I sat down, too confused to be exhausted. I had two more circuits to go for my first workout.

"What about that?" I asked, pointing at a man who held a bar in both hands and was busy shrugging his shoulders toward the sky.

"Oh that. That's for the trapezius muscles. I think 'traps' look unsightly on a man," Austin sniffed.

I noticed that none of the men by the machines had them. On the far side of the room, though, everyone did. These "traps" bunched up like single grapefruits on either side of the neck. They were thoroughly intimidating. I couldn't wait to get them.

"Anyway, I've just taught you the basics. For every exercise, there are tons of variations. You'll see as you go along."

Just then, a man dressed in a singlet and what appeared to be a tutu broke from the line for the deltoid press to introduce himself to me.

Quickly, Austin pushed him away, hissing, "Back off, Mary. He's mine!" The man skulked back to his station.

I couldn't let this go on any longer. "Is this a gay gym?" I asked.

"Look, honey," he replied. "*All* gyms are gay."

I examined the men by the machines. There Austin seemed right. "But what about them?" I asked, pointing to the free-weight lifters.

Austin laughed out loud. "*Especially* them," he said. "They just don't know it yet!"

I thanked Austin for the circuit and the information, and, as gently as possible, told him that I didn't think I'd be needing a training partner for the rest of the workout.

As he walked disconsolately back to his friends, I set about mastering the machine. "Joy and fierceness," I reminded myself, "joy and fierceness." I adjusted the weight so that I could accomplish the mandatory 12 repetitions. Invariably, I began pumping them out with ease, imagining the day I would walk unmolested through the streets. But before long, I was whimpering and hideously contorting my aching body as I pushed the last few up.

The men by the machine eyed me warily. I could sense it. I was doing something wrong. No one else at the machines seemed even to be trying.

Austin came over. "Take it easy," he whispered, "don't get into such a flap. Remember, Rome wasn't built in a day." But his words meant nothing to me. After jerking and bouncing my way through two more circuits, I silently congratulated myself—I was already one of the stronger men on that side of the room. I left the weight room flushed with victory.

My euphoria lasted all of 15 seconds, the time it took for Austin to find me back at my locker. He invited me to accompany him back to his place for a shower and a liver-and-whey shake. He had some slides he wanted me to see: some of the world's most famous bodybuilders in a variety of interesting poses. It was all part of "the lifter life-style," he assured me.

As politely as I could, I declined. Nothing more could happen, I thought, not on my first visit to the gym. After all, within the last two hours I'd suffered public humiliation, physical attack from a double amputee, and sexual harassment.

I breathed a sigh of relief and headed for the shower. That's when I heard him. He was no ordinary shower warbler.

"ONE, TWO, THREE, FOUR, FIVE, SIX, SEVEN!" the shout rang out, acoustically amplified by the shower tiles.

Bewildered, I looked at a man shaving at a nearby sink.

"Your first time, right?" he asked.

I nodded.

The man gestured with his head toward the shower. "They call

him 'The Counter.' Some say it was 'Nam, others he lost heavy on
Black Monday in Wall Street. Any case, the light's on upstairs, but
nobody's home."

I peeked in and saw him, alone, under the showerhead. He wore
a showercap, but the water wasn't on. It must have been on at some
point, though, because he was lathered with soap, and rubbing what
was left of the bar into his skin. Again, the voice boomed forth:
"ONE, TWO, THREE, FOUR, FIVE, SIX, SEVEN!"

Hearing my steps, he turned to face me. I looked down. No,
he wasn't visibly excited. That wasn't it, then. I gazed at his face.
Underneath the comedy of the shower cap, he looked utterly
haunted.

He bit his lip for a second, examining me. I waited, uncertain
yet for what. Tears, perhaps, or bitter, accusing words. Instead, his
eyes turned inward and he took up his recitation again, this time
louder than ever.

"ONE, TWO, THREE, FOUR, FIVE, SIX, SEVEN!"

It had been a long day, but as I showered all I could think about
was my next workout. Despite everything—the humiliation, the
harassment, the methodical man beside me—I was hooked. Standing insensate under that showerhead, none of it seemed to matter
very much. In the end, to my joy, I felt numb.

3.

THE WALK

I INVENTED, MORE OR LESS, MYSELF.

—*ION TIRIAC*

From that first night of September 1984 to March of 1985 I labored three times per week in the weight room. Every bar I pushed, every cable I pulled, moved me that much closer to a body weight of 200 pounds, to safety out on the street, to isolation. My fellow gym members watched, astonished by the obvious and frightening fact that this lifting was of crucial importance to me. None of the men by the machines understood the depth of my desperation.

There was a beautiful simplicity about it. I pushed the iron, and my body grew. The harder I worked, the better I felt. My routine brought order amid chaos. I knew just where to shuffle and when: Deltoids followed pecs, hamstrings followed quads. Always 12 reps, always three circuits. I barely paused between exercises, moving from station to station, cable to bar. And if I wasn't that strong, I could make up for it by continuing to exercise long after others had padded off to the showers. Set after set after set. Ninety minutes straight. Week after week. The training sessions passed in a blur. I put on 15 pounds in the first six months (bringing my weight up to 185) and regained my health. By March, my arms measured 15 inches, my neck 15½, my calves 15, my thighs 24, my chest 40, and my waist 34. I was on my way.

Still, one thing was bothering me. Despite my gains, things did not let up out on the street. Three-card monte sharps still took one look my way and rushed to set up shop beside me. My friend Jerry still lit up as I approached the subway escalator. And the general panic still followed me wherever I went. As much new armor as I had, I realized I would need a hell of a lot more.

Across the room lay the answer. Free-weights. The hugest men I'd seen, the men in the magazines, were always pictured with free-weights. They never seemed to trifle with the Universal. I couldn't imagine them encountering the slightest difficulty out on the streets. I had to break the plane.

At the edge of the crowd on the far side of the weight room, I saw him again. His upper body wasn't impressive, nor was his height. He stood as tall as my elbow. But his legs were enormous, the knees and ankles fairly drowning amidst the overhanging muscle. Noticing my stare, he put his dumbbells down and, rigid as a robot, walked over to me.

"I vomit the most. That's why my legs are the best," he said, in a high-pitched, girlish voice.

"The Portuguese Rambo," he proclaimed, extending his shaved forearm in my direction. He was completely bald, black, and about forty years old. He wore a sweatband on his head tilted at a rakish angle. His weight-lifting belt said BAD in black block letters.

"Hell, man, you can't build a house on a weak foundation," he said, pointing to his legs with an index finger. The words were familiar. I struggled to place them.

He shook loose the muscles of his massive legs, and we both watched the flesh flap like a loose sail in the wind.

"This here's the greatest sport, see, you work hard, you get rewarded." Familiar words again—where had I heard them before?

I nodded. I had witnessed his temper that first night; I didn't so much as utter a peep.

"See, we been watchin' you at the machines. And you know, man, we don't get it. Wha'choo want to work so hard for and waste it on them machines?" he asked, adjusting his groin with a public flourish. "Look, you want a chest bigger than Dolly Parton, right? Then follow me to the bench press."

It was what I'd been waiting for. At last, the breach to the free-weight group. I kept my head down and tried to drift in as inconspicuously as possible. Unsettling snatches of conversation from strange new voices floated around me.

"It was so dry, man, I had to crowbar it in. Once I got going,

like sandpaper. Man, it was music to my ears. She loved it too,"
one man whispered, lasciviously, to his friend.

Another thundered beside me: ". . . so I nailed him, twice, with
an uppercut. Should have seen his teeth there on the sidewalk. Like
bloody Chiclets. You don't mess with a *lifter*, man. . . ."

I hurried to the bench press where Mousie, The Portuguese
Rambo, was loading up a solid steel bar with 45-pound black iron
plates. Olympic Barbell Company, the weights said. The bar rested
on a trestle attached to the bench. By the time Mousie slid three
plates on each side of the bar, it sagged on either end.

"Three hundred fifteen pounds, man," Mousie said, lying with
his back flat on the bench. He did two repetitions, hoisting the bar
off the rack to arm's length, then bringing it down to touch his
chest before pushing it back up.

Mousie removed a plate from either side and let me try. This
wasn't a machine, and I knew it instantly. It was twice as hard as
what I had grown used to. I had no problem repping the 225-pound
weight; I had a grave problem balancing it. The bar listed like a
doomed ship in my hands.

"No problem, man, I'm here to spot you," Mousie said from
above my head.

With his fingers occasionally guiding the bar, I managed 10
repetitions. When I rose, unsteadily, to my feet I saw Bert eyeballing
me. Mousie recognized my fear.

"Relax, man," he said. "Bert's seen how hard you work out. He
really likes you. If he didn't, you would have found a Kotex in yo'
locker long time back, believe me." He prepared the bar again for
his next set.

"Besides, homeboy," Mousie added, rising from the bench when
he finished, "you don't come to the weight room to make friends,
you come to make gains." That too seemed familiar. Was it the
magazines? The Schwarzenegger canon?

After seven sets of bench presses, Mousie puffed out his chest
and walked with his shoulders held high to the incline bench. It
was slanted at 45 degrees and, he said, would work our upper
pectoral muscles.

Mousie grabbed a pair of dumbbells weighing 80 pounds each. He rested them first on his thighs, then took a deep breath, sat back on the incline, hiked the weights up to his chest, and pushed them to the sky 12 times.

I didn't understand it. My normal route back at the machines was to follow the line to the shoulder machine. Why more chest?

Mousie laughed between reps. " 'Cause we're workin' chest, man," he answered. "I already done back this mornin'."

"I thought you had to give your body a rest?" I asked, confused.

"You do, and the way you do it is to work a different body part every time, never repeatin' the same part the next day. See, it's called a 'split routine,' that is, workin' different muscles on different days, splittin' up yo' body parts."

As Mousie explained it to me, he was actually engaged in a "double-split" program, meaning twice-a-day workouts. He'd done back that morning, and would do chest that night. The next day, quads in the morning, hamstrings and calves that night. The day after that, shoulders in the morning, arms at night. The fourth day, or "off day," was reserved for rest. The entire program was called "three on, one off, double-splits," and, as I discovered, everyone in the free-weight section adhered to it.

"Why you think we don't look like them sorry-ass motherfuckers?" he asked, pointing to the men by the machines.

Again, I used half Mousie's weight. As I did my repetitions, I spied Sweepea lumbering through the door. He was the man I'd seen Mousie strangle six months earlier. They were the best of friends, I'd discovered, though Mousie frequently called him "The Missing Link" behind his back.

At five foot ten, Sweepea weighed 250 pounds. Of that bulk, an equal proportion was fat and muscle. He sported a Prince Valiant haircut, so shellacked with hair spray it looked like a helmet. Perched on the helmet was a black pirate's cap with a Jolly Roger emblem. All this, plus a missing front tooth. Smiling, he looked cherubic. Scowling, like a very bad dream.

Catching sight of Mousie, he bustled over to join us. When he spotted me, though, he slowed down, walking with exaggerated muscle-bound difficulty, as if he were fighting a torrential gale.

"What day is it, Mousie?" he asked.

"Monday," I interjected, trying to get at least something right. Sweepea eyed me with disdain.

"No," Mousie said, laughing. "Sam don't understand yet. It's chest and back today, Pea. Wha's it for you?"

"Legs," he groaned. This, I found, was the universal builder's reaction to "leg day," since the leg muscles were by far the most taxing to train.

"Look, you want to join us for chest?" Mousie asked, rolling his eyes at me. I gathered Sweepea would do anything to avoid a leg workout.

"Where are you?"

"Fourth set, second exercise," Mousie said.

Without a warm-up, Sweepea snatched up the 80-pound dumbbells and erupted in a burst of violent reps. I watched him in alarm as he screamed "Fuck Arnold!" at the top of his lungs, snorting and cackling at every repetition. I looked around me. None of the other free-weight men, too busy bragging among themselves or brooding individually on benches, paid him the slightest attention.

Without missing a beat, Sweepea finished, handed me my dumbbells, and said, now calm as a country pond, "Your set, man."

With my tongue between my teeth, I did the exercise, but timorously, spending as much energy balancing the weights as pushing them. At the eighth rep, I heard myself groaning and tried to stifle the sound.

Sweepea looked at me sadly and turned to Mousie. "He needs an attitude adjustment, man."

Mousie, taking his turn with the dumbbells, agreed. "Bro, you need to *attack* the weights, conquer the motherfuckers."

"That's right," Sweepea added. "You ain't with the sheep no more," he said, motioning to the men by the machines, "so stop bleating like one."

Sweepea emphasized his point by walking with his dumbbells to a sign on the wall that said:

PLEASE REPLACE WEIGHTS
TO RACK AFTER USE.

Directly beneath this sign, looking back at me, he dropped them dramatically from his shoulders to the floor.

"Quigs will come, man," Mousie said in warning. I gathered he meant Mr. Quigley.

Sweepea sucked in his gut and puffed out his chest. "Let him come, you see me quiverin', bro'? He turned his face slightly to the side and adjusted his pirate's cap.

That's when it hit me. Bad theater. Every word they uttered, every move they made seemed rehearsed—as rehearsed, in fact, as any performance I'd ever seen on stage. That explained the pregnant pauses before delivering the lines I knew so well from the magazines. Lines like "You gotta stay hungry," or "You work hard, good things will happen." Much of being a bodybuilder, I gathered, meant playing at being a bodybuilder.

Was this the essence of the sport? My reading seemed to confirm it. Since the first AAU Mr. America contest in 1939, bodybuilding involved premeditated reinvention. You chose who you wanted to be, and acted accordingly. So Angelo Siciliano picked up a dumbbell and became Charles Atlas. So Arnold Schwarzenegger became, for a time, Arnold Strong. If it was all a matter of role-playing, that explained Mousie's vision of himself as The Portuguese Rambo and Sweepea's pirate's hat.

It also explained my presence in the gym. The threat wasn't just from without, it also came from within. The fright I'd felt on the streets of New York I also felt deep within myself. Who was this man who cried not just at graduations and weddings but during beer and credit-card commercials? Who was this man terrified of his own rage, his own anger, his own greed, his own bitterness? Who was this man who never heard a compliment without hearing a subtextual insult, who never said "I love you" without resenting that other fact: "I need you." I couldn't deny it was me, or could I? There wasn't enough pomade, mouthwash, deodorant and talc in this world to eradicate my sins, but what if I created a shell to suppress them? What if my armor not only kept the world out, but kept me in?

I was more than willing to play the role of a builder if it could save me from myself. Sweepea and Mousie had found a disciple in their midst.

"No more Jell-O, ma!" I brayed, attacking the weight, as my new training partners broke into grins. During my reps, I resorted to what Schwarzenegger likes to call "The Arnold Mental Visualization Principle," more commonly known as the imagination, and saw my chest growing to such gargantuan proportions that no shirt on earth could contain it.

We went from incline presses to the decline bench, dumbbell presses to dumbbell flies, attacking our chests from every angle. Only two moves work for the chest, Mousie explained: a standard push movement from your nipples forward, and a standard fly movement, from arms outstretched at your sides to a position straight before you. Every chest movement is a variation of these two themes, and each theme involves the same principle: stretch (and by stretching, tear the muscle) and squeeze (flex it, contract it, during the whole movement).

At the end of the 90-minute workout, I had done so much stretching and squeezing, I could barely move. The free-weights had made all the difference. My chest spasmed and cramped back at my locker. It was caught in a state of shock. In circuit training, I was used to thirty sets per workout, but broken down into three sets per body part and ten different body parts. But tonight, we'd done thirty sets for just chest alone. The welcome onset of numbness was the only relief from the pain.

"God ain't exactly helped you with genetics, bro'," Mousie said, when I peeled off my tank top.

Sweepea pinched and prodded my aching body. He delivered his verdict with a sad shake of his head. "He's an ecto, man. That's tough."

I felt thoroughly defeated. I recognized the term from the magazines. They were filled with geneticspeak, classifying every human being into three basic body types: endomorphs, the naturally obese; mesomorphs, those born stocky and muscular; and ectomorphs, the lanky and bony. According to bodybuilding lore, you can change the way you look through weights, and racial stock might be taken into consideration (with advantages to Italians, Germans and Blacks), but of the three basic body types, ectomorphs have the most problems gaining muscle mass. For sheer size, they have the most to overcome. It wasn't what I wanted to hear.

"Arnold was an ectomorph," I proffered hopefully.

"Hey, Arnold was a *German*," Sweepea countered.

Again, my shoulders sagged. Mousie detected my misery. He asked if Sweepea and I would join him for a drink.

"Bodybuilders drink beer?" I asked.

"Milk is for babies. Arnold drinks beer!" they both shouted in what I took to be Austrian accents. Laughing uproariously, they revealed that they had seen the movie *Pumping Iron* again recently and were just quoting Arnold.

As we made our way to the bar on Fifty-second Street and Second Avenue, we ran into a man who looked as if he had sprung live right off the pages of my magazines.

He certainly didn't resemble anyone from the Y, free-weight section or not. He had achieved the look gained only by the most advanced builders. While my body was a mess of straight edges and right angles, his, so preposterously muscled, was a mass of curves, fleshy ellipses and ovals. They made his joints look tiny, and, in contrast to the great gobs of muscle, almost dainty.

He swept by us without a glance, not even acknowledging Mousie and Pea as iron brethren.

"That dude's got some *serious* muscle . . . " Sweepea said beneath his breath. "Bet he can bench four and squat five."

That much gym slang I knew. Sweepea estimated that a body like that could bench press four hundred and squat five hundred pounds. No one in our gym could do it.

"He's paid his dues, sure enough," Mousie added. As I was to learn, that was the greatest compliment one bodybuilder could pay another.

"He ain't no barbody, tha's for damn sure," Sweepea murmured.

"What's a barbody?" I asked, craning my neck for another look at the huge man. From a distance now, all I could see were the trademark signs of a builder: the simian, sloping shoulders, the V-shaped torso, the tiny waist.

"You know, all chest and arms, to impress the women up and down the bar. I seen loads of 'em at work. They just build those muscles you see in a Polo shirt. They don't got legs, or calves or nuthin'," Sweepea explained.

"Bet he's on the juice," Mousie whispered.

"Yeah? Well, I ain't asking him," Sweepea said fearfully.

"The juice?" I asked.

Sweepea smiled. "Yeah, man. You know, 'roids, shit, steroids."

"That doesn't seem very natural," I said. I'd noticed that the magazines were decidedly silent on that subject.

Sweepea looked at me with a wry grin. "What's natural?" he asked. "Looking at you, you think it's natural to go someplace and read for hours at a time. See, the way people think, that's OK 'cause you're developing your mind. Well, I say, what's wrong with developing your body? I mean, shit, who would *you* rather look like, Carl Sagan or Lou Ferrigno?"

I didn't reply. I was too angry and ashamed. After all, I wasn't the one walking up Second Avenue wearing a pirate's cap atop a Prince Valiant haircut. As for the shame, I knew that Sweepea was right; even strapped in my weight-lifting belt, I looked much more like Professor Sagan than like a builder. I felt that the last six months had been a waste.

At the bar, people stopped drinking and stared as we hit the door. A fire hydrant, a human avalanche, and me. Mousie and Sweepea, acknowledging the crowd, milked it, striding up to the bar in muscular, freeze-frame fashion.

I perked up with my first sip. After all, I had started free-weights, a triumph in itself. And after all my reading, I finally faced the real McCoy: bodybuilders. According to bodybuilding great Franco Columbu in his autobiography *Coming on Strong*, there are only two kinds of bodybuilders: the smart and the very smart. The magazines and the canon concurred. The time they didn't spend lifting, the iron press said, they spent writing violin concertos or poring over abstruse physics manuals, just for the fun of it.

I had to find out for myself. First off, how did these two support themselves? No trust fund babes, these.

"I'm a painter, man," Mousie said with dignity.

I was impressed. The builder as polymath. So far, so good.
"Landscapes?" I asked. "Portraits?"

"No, banks mostly, some supermarkets." He calmly sipped his
beer. "Just give me a ladder and a brush, and I'll give you a good
coat."

"I'm a crowd control engineer," Sweepea cut in. I looked puzzled.
"A bouncer," he explained. "I work downtown, nights mostly. Sometimes solo, sometimes in a team." A pause; then, predictably enough,
it came.

"But my job don't mean nuthin', man. I live to lift . . ." Sweepea
said. My two new friends clasped each other's hands above the table
in celebration of the delivery.

"Is that how you lost your tooth, on the job?" I asked Sweepea.

"Hell no, my father did that," he said, "back when I was a kid."

"I'm sorry," I muttered, embarrassed. "Do you get along better
now?"

Sweepea let loose with a great gap-toothed smile. "Yea, a *lot*
better. See now, *I'm* the man. He don't so much as say 'boo' without
askin' my permission. I give him an allowance, and he stays in his
room. You should see him now," he chuckled. "You think *I'm* missing
teeth. . . ."

"My job's cool, but it's temporary, understan'," Mousie spoke.
"Jus' give me five years, I be openin' up my own boutique. You know,
clothes and shit. So I gotta keep the flesh firm, man, that way, I
be advertisin' my goods just walkin' to work each mornin'."

As for Sweepea's future, he told me, with a faraway look in his
eye, before I could ask: "Sweepea's Gym, man, right out there in
Metro Park," he said, waving his hand before him.

Mousie turned to me. "What about you, man? What's the future
hold for you?"

They watched while I drew the image of a body on my cocktail
napkin. I gave no thought to genetics or racial stock. I set my
imagination free. The enormous chest and back tapered into a wasp-
sized waist. The legs flared out at the thigh. The calves looked like
footballs. Benching four and squatting five would not be a problem.
I spun the napkin around.

"You want to look like *that?*" Sweepea asked, incredulous.

Again, the pregnant pause. This time Mousie said it: "Then you best be prepared to make the necessary adjustments."

"What adjustments are those?" I asked, nervously shifting in my seat.

"Whatever adjustments are necessary," they intoned together, ominously.

First off, I would have to start eating five meals a day, plus special protein milk shakes. Then, I would have to adopt the double-split, three on, one off exercise program. It meant twelve workouts per week instead of three, thirty-five meals a week instead of twenty-one. It meant the purchase of a blender, a dietary scale, a caloric food encyclopedia. It meant a liberal supply of amino acids, vitamins, minerals. It meant purchasing wrist straps and knee wraps. But above all, they said, it meant "The Three D's."

"The Three D's?" I asked.

"The Three D's, bro'. You got to learn 'em, live 'em, lift wid 'em," Sweepea said, taking a swig of his beer.

Mousie nodded sternly. "Dedication, Determination, Discipline. That's bodybuilding," he said.

Half puritanism, half P. T. Barnum—it certainly did sound like bodybuilding. The training list was endless and involved everything. Everything, that is, save women. But what about women? I saw them in the magazines, wearing conveniently torn leotards and tights while they trained, but never in our gym. How could they have a place in a world that revered only ultimate muscle size and power?

"Hey," Mousie said, with a wicked leer. "You talkin' 'bout women? Well, there be a time and a place for everything."

"I had a girlfriend once," Sweepea said wistfully. "But I had to let her go. She couldn't even 'spot' me in the gym, so, you know, what's the point?" Mousie shook his head in sympathy. For Sweepea I gathered.

I changed the subject. "What led you to the gym, Sweepea?" I asked.

"Flippers," he said caustically, adjusting his pirate's cap. "I was skinny for my age, see, and my fifteenth birthday, my dad gave me flippers. 'What's these?' I says to him. It's not like we got a big pool in our backyard there or nuthin'. 'Them's flippers,' he says, 'to keep your bony ass from disappearin' down the drain when youse takes a shower.' He said it there, right in front of mommy. I been trainin' ever since."

I too had started bodybuilding as a matter of survival, I said. I asked them if they'd heard the latest statistics. There were approximately 300,000 violent crimes a year in New York City, 12,000 on the subway alone, the papers reported. Study after study had shown that "fear of crime" was the primary concern of New Yorkers. I needed a helmet in this tough town, I said. Hence the gym.

Mousie and Sweepea were strangely silent. I decided to make one last toast.

I raised my glass. "To survival!" I cried.

They uttered not a word. At some point, I'd said something wrong.

Finally, Sweepea spoke. "We're not talking about survival here. Hey, *cockroaches* survive. No, what we're talkin' 'bout is different."

"Yeah, you see, now you one of us. That mean you got *responsibilities*," Mousie explained.

I didn't get it.

"See, Hoss, you don't talk the talk, unless you walk the walk," Sweepea said firmly.

I still didn't get it.

It was apparent from his expression that Mousie had never before encountered anyone so dense.

"Look, you be a builder, you *carry* yo'self like a builder."

Sweepea and Mousie exchanged a glance and abruptly rose from the table. After hastily paying for the drinks, I followed them out into the night. And there it was, out on Second Avenue between Fifty-second and Fifty-third, that Mousie and Sweepea taught me "the Walk," that peculiar weight-lifters' waddle.

I'm sure you know it. The huge man we spotted the previous hour had done it particularly well. It's the not-so-secret signal among the iron cognoscenti of the presence of a dues-paying member of the bodybuilding guild.

I watched as first Sweepea, then Mousie strutted down the street. They swept their arms out to the side, as if the sheer massivity of their lat wings necessitated it. They burrowed their heads slightly into their shoulders to make their necks appear larger. They looked bowlegged, absurdly stiff, and infinitely menacing. At the corner light, they stopped and turned.

"Go on, now," Mousie said, encouraging me.

Fledgling builder that I was, I followed. I too jutted my arms out from my sides, keeping my elbows on the same line as my shoulders. I too carefully walked with my legs spread far apart to prevent the horrors of inner-thigh chafing from the immense size of the quadriceps.

I utilized The Arnold Mental Visualization Principle and imagined myself an itinerant pillbox. Safe behind my muscle walls, nothing could touch me as I awkwardly perambulated forward.

"No, goddamnit, that ain't it. You cowering!" Mousie shouted by the street light. "No wonder people mess wi'choo!"

"Like this, man, like this," Sweepea said, strutting down the street with his chest and shoulders held high, a trace of disdain on his lips.

Mousie watched Sweepea's swagger. "That's right, homeboy, with dignity, *dignity!*" he yelled.

At last, I understood. The Walk wasn't an upturned drawbridge and moat; it was a twenty-one gun salute, a full military cavalcade. I ran back down the street and tried again, this time curling my lip into a sneer. Once more, I used The Arnold Mental Visualization Principle, but this time I was Paul Bunyan, crushing Wisconsin hamlets with every giant step.

Deep in my reverie, I barely heard their shouts. "That's it, man, a positive mental attitude! You got it, now! You fine!"

"That which doesn't kill you makes you stronger!" I eagerly cried.

It was an expression I'd picked up in the weight room and the magazines. I found myself frequently using it of late as a substitute for "Have a nice day."

Sweepea and Mousie were delighted. From the corner of Fifty-second Street, the three of us parted that night after lengthy and elaborate soul shakes. Mousie headed due north for the South Bronx, Sweepea west to Metro Park. And I, I did "the Walk" all thirty blocks north by northeast back to my sublet.

4.

THE METAMORPHOSIS

*I'M JUST GOING TO KEEP RIGHT ON BUILDING.
YOU DO THE BEST YOU CAN TO STOP IT.*

—ROBERT MOSES

It was my father, the Ivy League Professor, on the line. I could almost smell his pipe. He sounded concerned.

"Dad, you're right. For a while there, I was genuinely fucked up. But everything's all right now, I'm really getting into bodybuilding," I crowed into the phone.

There was dead silence on his end of the line.

"Dad?"

I could hear him breathing slowly. Finally, he spoke. "September. The American Studies Program at Yale for your doctorate. You haven't forgotten, have you?"

Silence, this time on my end of the line. The fact was I'd so immersed myself in iron of late that it was the summer already, and I hadn't even completed the application.

My father's voice broke through. "Son, have you given any thought as to who your peers will be in this seamy enterprise?"

For five full minutes I defended my action. I mentioned democracy and deadlifting, "urban dissonance," and diarrhea. I spoke of falling air conditioners and of Jerry. I proudly described my new training partners, The Portuguese Rambo and Sweepea. I thought he would understand. He didn't. He was even more disgusted than usual.

"Yes, I can see it now," he said. "My son the bodybuilder, out on the streets of New York City with the rest of the poseurs of that particular metropolis."

"No, Father, believe me, it's not like that!" I blurted out. He didn't believe me.

I could hear the effort it took to keep his voice calm and measured. "Look, go ahead, go join the lepers—they're your limbs, after all. But do us all a favor, just don't tell your mother. Spare her the heartache for once, all right?" Then he hung up.

But it was too late—my mother already knew. A family friend from Princeton had spotted me on Fifty-ninth Street the previous week doing "the Walk." She had rushed to a nearby pay phone to give my mother a full report.

I armed myself with Sweepea's tape of the movie *Pumping Iron* and brought it over to my mother's apartment on my next "off day."

"Well?" I asked at the end, flushed myself. I always found the movie so inspiring.

Her face was like stone. "It's disgusting. These men have tits," she said.

"That's development, Mother. These men are engaged in the pure pursuit of physical development."

"Yes, and meanwhile they're functionally illiterate. One of them can't even speak."

"That's Lou Ferrigno, Mother, and it's not his fault. He's deaf."

"Well, you're not deaf, so why do you want to do this to yourself? And the bully with the gap between his teeth? Who is this punk? He's a moron."

"That's Arnold Schwarzenegger. He writes books."

"Not without a ghostwriter, he doesn't," she said.

I gave my mother a brief synopsis of Arnold's career. The fist-fights, the bodybuilding titles, the marriage. The sheer chutzpah of the man. To live without apology, without complaint, without compliance. And to think, as he wrote in his autobiography, he owed it all to bodybuilding. I did a quick flex with my bicep to assist my argument.

At this, my mother sunk her head into her hands. She sighed. She searched for words. Finally, she reached out and took my hands in hers.

"Look, son, I know the divorce has been hard on all of us, but don't you see? You're *internalizing*. You're punishing yourself. It's not your fault, really it's not. Look, I'll talk to Professor Levy at CCNY. I know he can still get you that job teaching freshman comp, OK?"

But I didn't hear her. My concentration was too great. She might have had my hands, but my calves were still mine, and I was flexing and unflexing them in time to the Mozart divertimento on her stereo. By the time she got to the NYU openings, I had quite a pump going.

When I left with Sweepea's tape under my arm, my mother stopped me at the door. She spoke urgently. "Please promise me one thing. Just don't tell your father. It would kill him."

Others, too, were raising objections to my new passion. In fact, I felt buffeted from all sides. Childhood friends called me in consternation. Apparently, my folly was so spectacular, so profoundly perverse, that even they had gotten wind of it. It was worse, somehow, than enlisting in the Marines or buying finger cymbals and joining the Hare Krishnas.

Fowler, an old college friend, met me for lunch. He wore his Phi Beta Kappa key; I wore a skintight tank top. Frankly, he was baffled. A sudden mania for single sculls would have been acceptable, he said. That, at least, had the imprimatur of Yale and Harvard behind it. But not this dark, dingy work, not this lifting. It was beyond comprehension.

I spent an interminable hour as he bombarded me with questions.

"Say, you weren't in a fraternity in college, were you? It's that, isn't it, the gym—some kind of weird brotherhood. Like Skull and Bones, right?"

"Hasn't it ever crossed your mind that this whole enterprise is rather *vulgar?* Is it your parents you want to hurt? Is that it? Is it your friends? Are you waiting for this to appear in the Alumni Notes? Goddamnit, why not do something with your life you can really be proud of?"

Fowler diagnosed my problem as a narcissistic personality disorder. He would have told me more, but he had to rush back to his job. He worked in public relations.

Only my gay friends were delighted. They thought they knew just where this would lead. A daily performance as studied and mannered as a bodybuilder's could only mean one thing. I *had* to be gay. They were planning a "coming-out" party, they said. All I had to do was give them the word.

Iron made sense to no one. To no one, that is, but me. All I knew was that I had found a sanctuary in the gym, and the more I trained, the better I felt. Out on the streets of New York, I'd found nothing but impediments, red lights, and stop signs everywhere. Inside the gym, I saw only green.

At dawn the workouts began, and always I wondered if I could recapture the glow, the magic pump I'd felt the previous night. I'd start slowly, warming up, testing myself, and then it would happen. Release. From exercise to exercise I'd go, feeling as if I were driving a car on a dark, wet night in the city. Suddenly, the stoplight just ahead turns green, the next one green, and green again. You don't need to brake for even one light. All you see is the road before you. You're not quite sure why, but you're going at the right speed at the right place and time. You take a quick look at the speedometer. Just to memorize the reading. But there's no need. Just keep it going, another light, another block, another weight, another exercise. Green, green, green.

Two hours each morning, two hours each evening, "three on, one off, double-splits." The gym was the one place I had control. I didn't have to speak, I didn't have to listen. I just had to push or pull. It was so much simpler, so much more satisfying than life outside. I regulated everything, from the number of exercises I performed each workout to the amount of weight I used for each exercise; from the number of reps per set to the number of sets per body part. It beat the street. It beat my girlfriend. It beat my family. I didn't have to think. I didn't have to care. I didn't have to feel. I simply had to lift.

With Mousie and Sweepea's aid and Arnold's canon as my guide, I worked out a program that emphasized the acquisition of "thickness." I wanted pure, unadulterated bulk. The striated slopes and gouged declivities of sculpted muscle could come later. Size first.

This meant eating, and lots of it. For breakfast, six poached eggs, six pieces of whole wheat toast, a whole grain cereal mix, a can of tuna. For my first lunch (around ten thirty), a pound of ground hamburger, a monstrous baked potato, a fistful of broccoli, a small salad. For my second lunch (two thirty), two whopping chicken breasts, spinach pasta, two slices of whole wheat bread. And dinner (eight thirty), dinner topped it all. Another pound of hamburger or steak, a super-size can of tuna, another potato, more bread.

It also meant drinking. In my case, in addition to a gallon of nonfat milk a day, three mammoth protein shakes—each one consisting of three raw eggs, three tablespoons of BIG protein powder, three teaspoons of lecithin granules (to lower the cholesterol level), a pint of nonfat milk, and a dash of vanilla (recommended by Arnold for flavor). With my meals and the shakes I drank between them, I was eating the equivalent of five six-course meals per day. And, just to be sure, I supplemented my meals with BIG Chewables. Each bottle contained 405 tablets filled with vitamins, minerals, and amino acids. I sucked and savored 108 of these tablets a day, the recommended dosage.

All the meals and the Chewables were ways to gain weight, and the way to make this weight stick was by working out in such a way that I actually lowered my metabolism. My "personalized program" emphasized the bench press, the deadlift, and the squat, the three major power movements in the gym. They also just happened to be the three most painful movements in the gym.

Under Mousie and Sweepea's care, I learned to wrap my knees, rise, and approach the squat rack "so angry you could spit tacks," as Mousie put it. Then, attacking the weight, I burrowed the back of my neck below the bar and ripped it off the rack, resting the whole weight just beneath my shoulders. From there, just a few steps backwards, and the squat began. Up and down, with two, then three, then four hundred pounds. And all the while, at six thirty A.M., the voices of my friends.

"BURY IT, MOTHERFUCKER!" they screamed. "BOTTOM OUT, YOU PATHETIC PIECE OF SHIT!"

According to Mousie and Sweepea, a squat wasn't a squat unless the squatter actually touched his calves to his hamstrings. Anything less, halfway down for instance, was labeled, disparagingly, "a football squat."

The squat was reserved for the dreaded "leg day," the bench press or, simply, the bench, for "chest day." But it was the deadlift, which I performed on "back day," which was the apotheosis of pain. The wrist straps (purchased by mail from The Monster Factory in

Connecticut) dangled from my wrists, until I bent down and wrapped them around the bar at my feet. At Mousie's nod, I surged upwards with my legs and back, keeping my ass down, rising with the weight until my back straightened and the bar rested on my upper thigh. The pain was unavoidable, a piercing sensation deep within my lower spine. Blood trickled from my scraped shins. Rep after rep, I grimaced and wobbled, while my training partners, arms folded across their chests, nodded their heads in approval.

The time I didn't spend working out or stuffing my shakes and meats down my gullet, I spent at the office slowly making my way to the medical unit on the fourth floor to check my progress on the Medco weight scale there. I say slowly, because Mousie and Sweepea had told me that to gain weight and lower my metabolism, I needed to eat more and move less. In fact, they said, slow down *all* extraneous movement. I gathered that extraneous movement meant any activity that did not involve the gym.

With all this food in my system, the transition from allegro to adagio was relatively easy. The hard part was keeping it all down. This was no easy chore considering my background. I had been raised in the "thin is in" neighborhood of Princeton, where madras-clad men starved themselves to impersonate Arrow shirt models. Too often, I found myself lunging for a streetlamp out on the street or lurching for the men's room at the office, to rid my guts of the wretched surplus.

But the bleeding and barfing I passed off as minor glitches in the overall program. After all, self-imposed pain seemed a significantly better alternative than the kind I witnessed out on the street, the kind issued by someone bigger, angrier, and meaner than his neighbor.

And besides, before my own eyes, I was growing. And the more I grew, the more I felt protected, *insulated* from everything and everyone around me. By September of 1985, I hit the 200-pound mark. Six months later I reached 220. I celebrated by changing my march to the Medco from a weekly to a daily event and taking time out from my typing for impromptu posing sessions in the men's room.

The bathroom was the only place on the floor full of mirrors,

mirrors I desperately needed to examine my form. The magazines constantly stressed the bad press mirrors and bodybuilding received, but it had nothing to do with vanity. Mirrors were simply a necessary tool for critical physique appraisal. Or so my books and magazines said.

But whenever I locked the door behind me and quickly peeled off my shirt, I had to stifle a wolfish whistle. How my beanpole figure had changed in the last year! Before, I'd been what body-builders call "skinny fat," which means a human boneyard covered in an opaque veneer of lard. But no longer—now as I flexed I saw veins larger than tug ropes spring up from nowhere to lace my biceps and triceps, now clearly delineated. My forearms, once celery stalks, were now bowling pins. Even my chest had changed. It was no longer completely concave.

Listening for approaching footsteps, I'd spend a few minutes "standing relaxed." Along with "the Walk," it is the most common form of bodybuilding presentation. It starts with a slight bend at the knees to make sure the quads look fuller. Then, an ankle shift with toes pointed outward for calf display. A spread of the latissimus dorsi, a resulting outward sweep of the arms, a lift of the shoulders, and there you have it. The position is really just a standing version of "the Walk." The trick is to flex and tighten all your muscles while maintaining an air of insouciance. Only the best builders can smile through the pose as their limbs begin to tremor and quake through minutes of rigid immobility.

"The crab," a far more dramatic pose, I saved for the cadenza. One of a number of "most-muscular" poses, the crab brings every-thing to the surface, making the crabber look like a human anatomy chart. I'd start with a deep breath, then, bending forward at the waist, fiercely thrust my arms before me like a crab's pincers and watch. The inevitable result was veins shooting like lightning across the skin of my chest and shoulders, muscle fibers dancing just be-neath my skin, my whole body shuddering. Bodybuilders call this veiny look "vascularity," and it is prized as proof that a builder can be huge without being fat. Just a few minutes after entering the men's room, I'd emerge purple from the exertion, not a bit sheepish, holding my chin higher than ever.

Though no one ever caught me crabbing, at work my muscular behavior became a cause of concern on the floor. It was the general consensus that I had gone too far. Way too far. Some could understand the need to "fill out," as I put it, and gain a few pounds. But two hour sessions in the morning and two more hours at night, five meals a day, vitamin supplements, and protein shakes?

And if that wasn't enough, well, there was the noise of my accouterments and the demands of my discipline. I installed an industrial-strength stainless steel blender in my cubicle for my shakes. I monopolized the floor's sole refrigerator for my meats and milk and eggs, and continuously worked the microwave for a fresh feeding.

My cubicle, which I renamed The Growth Center, became a depot for desiccated beef liver tablets, multivitamin packs, bag after bag of branch-chain amino acids, cartons of Carboplex (a carbohydrate concentrate), and protein powder. What with the magazines and the canon scattered across the floor, the whole place was a muscle minefield, but I didn't see it that way, not then. Not when I was caught in the full raging force of "the disease."

Oh, I knew I was afflicted all right. I studied who and what I was every day in my magazines and in the mirror. My research helped to explain to curious coworkers why, though I lifted weights, I didn't look like the 350-pound Russian lifter Vasilly Alexeev. There are actually three distinct groups of weight lifters: Olympic lifters, of which Alexeev was one of the greatest; powerlifters; and bodybuilders. All of them worship iron, but each in their own way, and they get along about as well as Catholics and Protestants in Northern Ireland.

Olympic lifters (the only one of the three weight-lifting activities recognized by the International Olympic Committee) compete in only two movements: the snatch, and the clean and jerk. They are simply two stylized means of propelling a weighted bar from the floor to overhead. Both require agility, speed, coordination, and strength.

Powerlifters, whose sport came into being in the early 1960s as an offshoot of Olympic lifting, compete in three different exercises: the bench press, the deadlift, and the squat (the three I had incorporated into my size program). Pure power works for the aptly named powerlifters. Coordination and agility are not at a premium.

The only thing Olympic lifters and powerlifters share in common is a judging system based wholly on the weights they lift. Bodybuilders are the sole group who are awarded points on such intangibles as charisma and tan (or competition color). Bodybuilders don't perform specific exercises with weights on stage for competition. They use the weights simply to change the appearance of their bodies. They're landscape architects, creating a mound here, a furrow there, as well as illusionists, positioning themselves in a certain manner on stage to their advantage. Bodybuilding requires some strength, a lot of endurance, and by far the most time spent in the gym.

In the competitions, bodybuilders go through "mandatories"—a set of mandatory poses—in the morning, where the judges compare the body parts of the builders. And then, in the evening the competitors return to perform a choreographed routine incorporating set poses and moves, the ones I practiced in the men's room.

At the office, visits from my dwindling number of friends on the floor became increasingly infrequent. The few times fellow workers did venture to The Growth Center I found myself capable of discussing nothing but lifting. While my friends talked about upcoming books and their college reunions, I sternly lectured them on the importance of "the three D's" and maximum protein utilization.

The real problem at work, though, wasn't my muscle homilies, my private posing, my pigsty of protein powder, my magazines, or my blender. No, the real problem was *me*. My physical metamorphosis had brought with it a completely different way of perceiving the world and my place in it.

Attitude is what separates the best bodybuilders from the also-rans, I learned (look it up, the heading *attitude* is directly under *arthritis, degenerative* in bodybuilding manuals). If you think of yourself as a person of consequence, then you are halfway toward achieving that distinction. If you don't think you can lift 400 pounds on a deadlift, then, believe me, you won't. Every magazine article I read made that crystal clear.

Mousie and Sweepea were right that first night. I *had* needed an attitude adjustment. And I don't know exactly when the transformation happened—all I can say is that it did. Without being fully aware of it myself, I became the kind of man I had once feared and despised. I became, in fact, a bully.

First, I changed my clothes. Out went the Oxford button-downs. They could no longer contain my bulk. From the back of the bodybuilding magazines, I sent off for XXL T-shirts specially cut for bodybuilders. Each day I'd wear a new one to work, only the emblems changed. One day, a lifter holding a sledgehammer, surrounded by inspirational bons mots like "Tough Times Don't Last. Tough People Do." Another day, a snarling Rottweiler, with the legend, "Don't Growl If You Can't Bite." Just eighteen months before, these shirts would have billowed over my bony frame. Now, they stretched over my mountains of muscle like a taut second skin. Thanks to my swelling quadriceps, my pants were so snug, I had to spend company time in the men's room applying baby powder to the skin of my inner thighs for cool relief.

Then, my manner of speech. It had been too tame before, too timid. No wonder I never got my way in life. I went from answering the phone meekly to shrieking "SPEAK!" into the receiver on the first ring. I learned to pause professionally in dramatic bodybuilding fashion during the delivery of my lines as did Sweepea and Mousie. And I lowered the pitch and timbre of my voice to the point where I could make a laundry list sound like The Constitution.

I perfected "the Walk" as well, roaming the aisles on forays from The Growth Center. By habit now, I made use of The Arnold Mental Visualization Principle, rolling through the deep as the great leviathan, watching the minnows scatter to their offices at my approach. From behind quickly closed doors, I could hear some gasp, and others murmur only "gross!"

I was no longer me. Gone was the cautious, passive, tolerant student, the gentle soul who had urged departing friends to "take care" and actually meant it. The new me was a builder. A builder who had no time for anything that wouldn't help him grow. Who, in place of the words "thank you," barked "no kindness forgotten, no transgression forgiven." As my behavior changed, the smiles of my fellow workers faded, their greetings tapering off to a nervous nod of the head. There was fear in the air.

It was all wonderful—for me, that is. Others on the floor, like Benny Potemkin, came to feel differently. Benny was an earnest manuscript editor who could never be found without his copy of *The Nation*.

"Be my guest," he said one day, opening a door for me.

As a builder, I accepted charity from no one. It was inconsistent with the concept of paying my dues.

"Not in a million years, my friend," I bellowed in my best builder's bass.

"I insist," Benny said.

A test of wills. I relished this. I just stood before the door and smiled. Wild horses couldn't drag me through. It was a stalemate. Neither of us would budge. So I relied on what I'd learned in the weight room, suddenly wrapping both of my arms around Benny, lifting him clear off the floor and catapulting him through the door.

He landed ingloriously on his ass and looked back in rage. "God damn you! You're fucking insane!" he screeched.

He rubbed his aching bottom, stood up and straightened his suit. Then he rushed off to the divisional president's office to lodge a formal complaint against me.

The writing was on the wall. For a moment, I panicked. But then I remembered Sweepea. "Dignity," I heard his voice saying, *"dignity!"*

I quit before they could fire me, strutting back to The Growth Center with chin and chest held high. I would not let this disturb my workout. Arms and shoulders, I believe, were on the agenda for the evening. I packed my things, the food, the blender, the meats, and left the office forever.

And wouldn't you know it, I ran into Jerry after work. Once again, he was haunting the subway platform, wearing his sandwich board. As soon as he saw me, he rushed over. First he ran his eyes over the blender and the bag of food in my hands. Then, he took in the rest of my body and stopped dead in his tracks. Faced with the new me—the muscles, the T-shirt, the glare—he balked. My heart soared.

The whole thing worked. If even Jerry could detect the ocean of violence raging just beneath my taut T-shirt, I was saved. The makeover was complete. I'd lost my job, but I'd found my way of life. At this point, I was far beyond recall.

5.

THE BUNKER

---

*IF I ELIMINATE EVERYTHING, HOW WILL I
EXIST? . . . WHAT HAPPENS IF YOU DROP ALL THE
THINGS THAT MAKE YOU I?*

—GRAHAM GREENE

I had always been told that to grow up meant to stop wanting those things you couldn't have. But everything I'd learned from bodybuilding taught me to fight this notion. You *can* become the person you dream of being, bodybuilders said. You *can* defy both nurture and nature and transform yourself. It's the essential drama of the dream, though in the end it might take more than you're willing to give.

But not me, I vowed. If it meant feeling safe and protected, I was willing to give up *everything*. Along with my job, I gave up my friends—my non-bodybuilding friends, that is. "As they say, if you stick around cripples—mental or physical—long enough, pretty soon you'll learn how to limp," Arnold counsels in *Posedown!* I took him at his word. Fowler telephoned, wrote, even knocked, but I didn't answer. Next, I surrendered my tony Upper East Side apartment. If I scrimped and moved to Queens, I wouldn't even have to work again. I could simply become a gym rat, serving time until I could get paid for using my muscles in some fashion.

Several years before, on my twenty-first birthday, I had inherited some money from my grandfather. At the time, my father had advised me to save it for something really important—a house, for instance, or eight years of graduate school. I now took him at his word and used it to finance my life as a bodybuilder. I called the move an investment in my future. My father (we were still talking then) called me psychotic.

I found the perfect spot in Sunnyside, Queens, just a few subway clicks from my gym in midtown Manhattan. "Cozy bachelor pad," the New York *Times* classified ads described it, but when the realtor, Mr. Tarantino, drove me to the house I got the feeling that I'd found much more than that. The only entrance was from the back, around a gate and through a storm door embedded in the ground. The basement steps led to another door, this one triple-locked and buried in the concrete foundation of the house.

It was love at first sight. My "cozy bachelor pad" turned out to be a storm cellar. There were no windows—anywhere. Not in the tiny bathroom, the even smaller kitchenette, not even in the first of my two front doors. The ceiling was barely six and a half feet tall, made even lower by a number of hanging steel pipes. Their function was a mystery until a family member upstairs flushed the toilet.

It was a real bunker, four concrete walls protected by earth in its outer perimeters and by the house above. And there were two refrigerators in the corner. Two! My heart skipped a beat in joy.

"I'll get rid of one of 'em for you," Mr. Tarantino assured me.

"Not on your life," I said, pausing out of habit now. It had become second nature. "I have need of two."

"Suit yourself," he said, shrugging.

"One more thing," he called at the door. "No telephone. You want I should call the company for installation?"

"No thanks." I smiled, checking the walls for an outlet for my blender. "No phone, no mail, nothing."

He looked at me searchingly, then stared at my check in his hands. He shrugged and clambered up the stairs out into the light.

A mattress, a lamp, an easy chair. I scavenged the neighborhood for discarded furniture. I liked to think of myself as Robinson Crusoe, marooned and forsaken by chance on a barbarous isle. Crusoe withdraws to his fortress, whose walls he creates with sharpened sticks. I withdrew to mine. Our situations seemed to me identical, and our reactions not dissimilar. The real difference lay in our methodology. His musket, my peaked bicep; his sharpened stick, my straining pectorals; his fortress, my bunker.

The reality of course was somewhat different. Far from the ship-wrecked Crusoe, I was a cosseted preppie who felt guilty enough about his own advantages to betray them and begin life again, from scratch. But the reality didn't matter; I was so far removed from it that my life pre-iron no longer existed for me. It had all happened to someone else, someone smaller, frailer, less substantial than this new-and-improved packaged version.

From what I could see in the gym, the best bodies were developed through consistent training, hard work, and attention to diet. Those who wanted the best bodies, and were willing to do whatever it took to get them, got them. It had nothing to do with slow-twitch or fast-twitch muscles, with "metabolic optimizers" or "the mind-body connection" touted by the latest article. The scientific jargon was just a veneer of respectability concocted by magazine editors to sell the product. In the same vein, Arnold labeled bodybuilding "progressive weight resistance training," a euphemism bringing to mind modern science and white lab coats rather than mirrors and the acrid smell of sweat.

But the articles were all nonsense. What mattered was sheer desperation and effort. And with that in mind, I felt I was anyone's equal. My idol wasn't a bodybuilder, but a coal miner: one Alexei Stakhanov of the Soviet Union. On August thirty-first, 1935, he drilled 102 tons of coal in six hours, fourteen times the norm for his shift. For his efforts, the word Stakhanovite was added to our vocabulary. Forget the science, just lift more than the norm during the shift.

So, twice a day, I emerged from the bunker and pounded away in the gym, two hours per session. And it worked. The bigger I got, the better I felt. By July of 1986, my weight rose to 230 pounds. I'd leave it to others to feel. I'd experience whatever physical pain was necessary to cauterize my real pain, the pain I felt in being so vulnerable, so assailable.

I stuck to the basic exercises in my routine, performing four or five per body part. On back morning, I started with pull-ups, which became increasingly difficult as I gained weight. Then, in my mass mania, on to the bloodletting of deadlifts, or, as an occasional substitute exercise, bent-over barbell rows. These were not as taxing as deadlifts, but they were painful enough so that I was the only gym member who actually did them. They are a kind of abbreviated deadlift, where you keep your knees bent slightly, torso parallel to the floor, then bring the barbell up with your arms and back muscles to touch your chest, then down to the floor again. I concluded my back workout with low pulley rows, the collegiate rower once more.

A return trip to the bunker for as many meals as I could hold down, then back to the gym for chest at night. I kept with the great mass producer, the bench press, working my upper chest, as I had with Mousie that first time, with dumbbell presses from an incline position, then flies and declines.

The next day, legs were an adventure all in themselves. Just mentally preparing for a leg workout was exhausting, since experience proved there was no way to avoid the pain. Once in the gym, I started first with the mass-gainers, as usual. In the case of legs, it was squats. Eight excruciating breathless sets in which I drowned the creaking noise of my knees and lower back with screams of effort. The leg-press machine followed squats. This movement simulated the squat, except that it changed the angle from a vertical move to a horizontal one. It wasn't as good for my muscles, but it was a hell of a lot easier on my joints. In conjunction, both worked well. The hack squat machine was next, the third angle of the morning in which I worked legs. Once again, the movement didn't change, legs to chest, legs locked, but the hack squat was set at an incline position. I adjusted a padded leather yoke over my shoulders connected to the weights, lowered myself to my haunches and up again, twelve times. I ended the session with five sets of leg extensions, the exercise designed to scoop cuts into the legs, and make startling divisions between the long vertical quadriceps muscles.

At night, I'd return for what we called "hams and calves," the second and final part of leg day. Stretch and squeeze, the same philosophy always applied, no matter which muscle I was working. I'd grab a barbell at thigh height, then, keeping my legs straight while bending my back, bring the weight down to my toes. These were stiff-legged deadlifts, basically, touching your toes with a 300-pound weight attached to your wrists. It was an exercise designed specifically for the hamstrings. The pain I felt in my lower back after doing a set made clear that every movement in the gym also, to some degree, works some other part of the body.

Leg curls followed stiff-legged deadlifts, performed on the Universal station, where I compared notes with my old friend Austin and the rest of the Universal gang. Then, without a break, on to calf blasting. Calf exercises are the only movements in the gym which, universally, bodybuilders find boring. Like the exercises for all other body parts, there are variations; you can bomb them from a standing position, from a seated position, with friends mounted on your shoulders and back, but it is tedious work. Even the pump isn't a reward in this activity, when it arrives it is so painful that most bodybuilders simply avoid the exercise altogether. But not me. From the moment I started lifting, I was all too aware of my calf deficiency. My solace was that it had once been a shortcoming for Arnold as well. He solved the calf crisis by cutting all of his long pants at the knee to expose the problem. Bodybuilding lore had it that he gained two inches in one year, working that much harder in the constant shame he forced himself to suffer. I emulated "The Austrian Oak" and used the scissors on my pants. I even rolled my socks all the way down to my ankles to emphasize the point.

And at night, I was merciless, blasting them beyond pain. I stepped up to a raised wooden block and bent at the waist. Up and down I'd go on my toes, trying to isolate the movement until only my calves moved. Then, I'd make like a horse, or as they call it in the gym, a donkey, and Mousie and the bulk of Sweepea would clamber astride my back for added weight. New angles, new pain; the seated calf machine by the window, the weights connected to a pad on my knees as I brought my toes up and down. I ended the marathon on the standing calf machine, the weight stack connected this time to my shoulders.

I learned to judge a successful leg day by the quality of cramping every evening. If I could fall asleep back at the bunker without severe muscular pain, then something was terribly wrong. While my legs spasmed through the night, I'd dream of Tom Platz, the so-called "Golden Eagle." More than any other bodybuilder, he'd given up everything to reverse the course of nature. He had been born with a miserable structure, his hips wider than a yardstick, his shoulders narrower than a ruler. But through sheer industry, through set after set of 315-pound squats for 50 straight reps, through training sessions interspersed with vomit and blood, Tom had hurdled these obstacles and become Mr. Universe. His thighs were each larger than an average human's waist. His calves looked like watermelons.

On the morning of the third day, inspired by my dreams, I sped to the gym for my deltoid exercises, movements specifically geared to accrete muscle in the front, middle, and rear sections of the shoulder. All bodybuilders strain for the look known as "cannonball deltoids." Arnold had them, Tom had them, and I wanted them. So I paid my dues at the shoulder-press rack.

From a seated position, I grabbed a loaded barbell behind my neck, brought it all the way up above my head to the point where my elbows locked out, and back down again. As my body weight increased, so did the weight I was pushing above my head. There are some bodybuilders who can press 315 pounds eight times or more behind their head. I wasn't one of them.

Lateral raises were next, where I picked up a pair of 40-pound dumbbells from the floor and, from a position by my hips, brought them up laterally until my stiff arms were straight on line with my shoulders. Five sets of 12 to 15 reps and on to the rear delt machine. This machine is normally used for the pectoral muscles, but through practice bodybuilders have found that if you face the machine instead of sit in it, you can actually work the back of your shoulders. I concluded the morning with Arnold presses, Arnold's signature move in the gym, a shortened shoulder press with wrist supination, or twisting, to work each head of the deltoid.

The third and final night was the easiest. There is not a bodybuilder alive who finds it difficult to work arms. The pump is practically immediate, the gains relatively easy and painless. I blasted my biceps with so-called "cheat curls," the standard power movement. Barbell in hands, I brought the weight up from my thighs to my chin. Sounds easy. With 135 pounds or more it's not. The first few reps I performed strictly, the last few I swayed my back and shimmied my hips, using any trick I could to get the weight up. Thus the "cheat." Seven sets later, I headed for stricter bicep exercises, like alternate dumbbell curls. The dumbbells enabled me to slow down the basic curl movement, first lifting one arm to my chest, then the other. Preacher curls followed, the exercise so named because the lifter positions his arms upon an inclined pad, grabs a weight, and strictly brings it up to his chin, at which point he looks like a supplicant of iron.

A quick drink at the water fountain and on to triceps, the backs of the arms. First a trip to the Universal and the cable push-down station. Knees slightly bent, weight just a bit forward, I grabbed the bar (connected to a cable attached to a weight stack) at my chest and brought it down to my thighs. The usual five sets, the usual 12 reps. Then, back to the bench press, this time not to work the mass of the chest, but the mass of the triceps. Just a minor adjustment to accomplish the variant exercise—bringing the hands in a few inches apart on the bar instead of at shoulder width. Finally, dips, in which I grabbed the two handles of a rack and lowered my body down, then up, down and up without touching my feet to the floor.

I never varied the exercises, only the way I did them. And the fact was: I had to vary the way I did them to keep from going completely insane. Lifting is more than demanding. It is fundamentally boring. Each day, you know exactly what you are going to do, so you have to incorporate new techniques or movements, however minor, to keep from counting staples in the walls or numbering the tiles on the ceiling.

So I ran the rack, starting with hundred-pound dumbbells on the incline press, getting as many repetitions as possible. Then, casting them aside, I reached for the 90's without a pause, more reps, on to the 80's, the 70's. By the time I reached the 30's, the rack was empty and my chest inflamed beyond pain.

And when I didn't run the rack, I resorted to other "intensifiers," like pyramids, strip sets, forced negatives, forced reps, anything. All of the variations fell under the principle of shocking the muscle, forcing it to work in a way it had never worked before. Thus I alternated exercises, some days doing 15 reps per exercise, other days 8, some days starting out on the first set with a high number of reps, then, gradually decreasing the number of reps as I added weight, until I went to lighter weight and higher reps again (the pyramid principle).

Forced reps involved Sweepea's sweating face inches from mine as he forced me to get more reps on a given exercise than I could without him. Sometimes this meant the touch of his finger on the bar, making it easier for me; sometimes, it meant a touch of his finger on the bar to make it harder (forced negatives).

Strip sets, "21's," "I go/you go," anything we'd heard of we used. It wasn't long before I was supersetting all of my exercises in the gym, dashing to complete one right after another without a second's rest. Two in a row, rest, two in a row, rest. You could combine another body part in the second exercise, or just add to a first to make it that much more painful. Bang, bang, bang, from exercise to exercise I'd go. And when I emerged, showered, shaved, and pumped each morning, I felt reborn.

The result was continuous, extraordinarily rapid growth—for me at least. Since I was the only one at the gym actually doing the lifting, I was the only one actually growing. Other builders clung to me like burrs, hoping that they'd make similar gains. But they didn't because no one trained like I did. No one else was willing to suffer this kind of pain. Not Sweepea, not Mousie, and, God knows, not Austin. I became the toast of the gym, closer than anyone to that magic land of "benching four and squatting five."

On my off days, I grew impatient, yearning to speed up time and start the next day's workout. The more I trained, the more desperately I needed to train. My body ached for the pump. I couldn't live without it, that burning sensation acquired through bombing a muscle area. At first it feels like someone rubbing heat balm on the particular muscle you're working, it feels almost numb; then the analgesic spreads. Within minutes, you feel your whole body glowing, as if you're the sole source of illumination in a dark world. You can't help but smile. And it was the pump that kept me going, endorphins running to the rescue whenever I called. If Sisyphus gets a pump from his eternal exercise, I assure you all this time he's been a happy man.

In just a year fellow lifters went from disparaging my genetic heritage to lauding it. It was the common consensus in the weight room that my parents must be German. Sweepea and Mousie, far from acting like jealous siblings, gloated like doting parents. "We've created a monster," they grew fond of boasting. I'd catapulted past them ages ago. Even Bert, the snarling gargoyle, had only smiles of admiration for me.

Now I not only looked like a builder, I acted like one in front of my friends. Sweepea and Mousie watched proudly when an iron neophyte made his way over to me at the end of my second year. He reminded me of myself—or at least that self I'd discarded two years earlier. Spectacles magnified his lemur eyes. His complexion was milky white, and he wore his high school gym shorts too high (closer to the nipples than the navel was not the current fashion).

Despite appearances, though, he had caught the disease. That was evident as soon as he snarled at himself in the mirror and did an agonizing high rep set of arm curls. It was apparent that he hated himself as he was. Just watching him was painful.

"My name's Joel," he said mournfully. "I was wondering, just what is it that you guys eat and drink to get so darn big?" His voice signaled pure desperation.

"Why," I pronounced, arching my back and raising my shoulders, "I would drink donkey urine from the source itself, if I thought it would make me grow. We all would. Damn it, man, we're body-builders!" I laughed heartily, turning to see Sweepea and Mousie break up themselves. Joel turned green. I dug my elbow deep into his sunken ribs to make sure he realized I was joking. "Just look for anything high in protein and low in fat," I explained.

My transformation was complete, outside and in. The builder persona was no longer a role—it was actually me. And though I no longer had a nine-to-five job, I hardly thought of myself as jobless. Just the opposite: Now I was a workaholic who devoted every hour of the day, one way or another, to the gym. Even professional bodybuilders train at most around 4 hours a day (Austin had been right; you can only do so much to build before you cross the line and break down the muscle tissue by doing too much), so the time I didn't spend actually lifting, I spent in support of or preparation for it.

I was at the supermarket stocking up on fuel to help me with my lifting. Roaming the aisles, I picked up each week 70 eggs, 14 tins of tuna, 10½ pounds of beef, 10 pounds of chicken, 9 gallons of nonfat milk, 4 loaves of bread, and as many sacks of brown rice, whole wheat pasta, baking potatoes, and fruit as I could load into my shopping carts (one wasn't enough).

Or I was back in the bunker, gobbling my daily multivitamin packets. I took 6,666 percent of the daily minimum requirement of vitamin B_1, 5,882 percent of B_2, 1,333 percent of E, 1,000 percent of C, and so on. I had more letters inside me than the alphabet, all to cover the rigors of training. I supplemented even my supplements with desiccated and defatted beef-liver tablets to help my liver and kidneys process the overload.

The lifting life meant laundry as well. Once a week, on my off-day, I did "the Walk," bags in hand, from the bunker to the corner laundromat. I monopolized a row of six washers for my jocks and sweatpants and T-shirts and tank tops and then six driers. Kerchiefed Queens mothers shook their heads in sympathy, assuming I managed a local Little League team.

Every few hours, no matter where I was, I found myself running through my muscle inventory, checking to make sure I was still there. From head to toe, I'd squeeze and flex every body part: traps? check; deltoids? check; pecs? check; lat wings? check; bi's and tri's? check; quads? check; calves? check. All present and accounted for.

The rest of the day I spent preparing muscle food or resting my muscles on the bed, mentally gearing up for the next muscle-fest in the gym. If I wasn't reading a muscle magazine, I was riffling through a new catalog from the neighborhood big man's clothing store, wondering what tent-sized finery I might use to outfit my muscles. Muscles, muscles, muscles.

An article I read haunted me. The piece had reported Schwarzenegger's happiness in signing a new movie contract. In it, Arnold said, "Arnold is back where he belongs, on top." I longed for that conviction, the ease and peace of mind that would come from the simplistic belief that there is a top and a bottom in this world. Top and bottom, black and white, good and evil, positive and negative, big and small, I retreated into the narrow world of dichotomy. I no longer had questions, only solutions, and they all pointed to the weight room.

So long as I was trussed in my weight-lifting belt, life was as neat and tidy as a crossword puzzle. I stopped thinking of my friend Eric by not thinking at all. Spotting a would-be suicide jumping into the Hudson River off a pier, Eric watched the crowd congregate above the man sinking in the water. The drowning man had an audience, and not one soul offered a hand to help. But Eric, new to New York, couldn't stand it another second. He dove off the pier, struggled through the murky water to reach the man and caught him. They went down together, the man's hands wrapped around Eric's neck. It took the police hours to find the bodies. As long as I lifted, I didn't think about the life Eric might have led. I didn't think about how my parents were no longer on speaking terms. I didn't think about my own sterile preference for concepts and ideals rather than people. I didn't recognize just how convenient it was for me to permit myself to love a woman who, because of her betrothal to another, couldn't return my part-time affection. I was ripe for the disease, all right.

I wasn't the only one afflicted. Silently, steadily, the disease had reached epidemic proportions: Not just in health clubs, but out on the street, on the ferry, in cafés, bars, public parks, even libraries. Wherever there were people, there were builders. Of course, "the Walk" was a dead giveaway. But there were other signs, more subtle but equally telling. The shaved and tanned forearm of a subway strapholder. The shock of swollen gastrocnemius muscles below a father's shorts in the grocery line. The bunched bulging traps of a bike messenger. All it took between us was a quick look, then a nod and a smile. We were not alone. Race, religion, nationality, they were inconsequential. First and foremost, we were bodybuilders—and we breathed easier because of it.

To complete my identity, I shaved my whole body. It was the sole remaining impediment to the way. Body hair obscures muscle definition (the cuts chiseled between distinct muscle groups) and separation (the striations and visible muscle fiber making up the separate parts within the muscle itself). I thought of it as just a way of seeing who I was.

As with steroids, the magazines avoided altogether the subject, since it included the disturbing matter of shaving the legs. But I gathered from Mousie and Sweepea that I would need a number of blades. So I bought my "Lady Bics," ten of them, retreated to the bunker and ran the bathwater.

I started with my upper body, lathering everything above the waist save for my head. Wrists first. Up my forearms, over my biceps, and around the hanging flesh of my triceps to my shoulders. Off it came, the hair from my chest, my abdomen, my underarms. As soon as one blade clogged with hair, I discarded it and swept up another. It seemed simple.

It was—until I stood up and tried my legs. I would have been better off using a machete. As soon as I began to pick up speed, my ankles and knees acted as vicious speed bumps to the razor's edge, sending the blade soaring over smooth plains only to halt and bite into one of my bony knobs. All in all, the whole thing took an hour and ruined ten good blades.

And when I rose from the tub and looked down at my naked form, I was amazed. It wasn't the body—it was the blood. I looked as if I'd run a full marathon through briars. I waited for the sharp shock of pain, but it didn't come. I didn't feel a thing. I was no longer connected to my own body. It had become simply an abstract concept, a shell to be polished and plucked with regularity.

When I was dressed, the scrape of fabric on my skin constantly served to remind me of the state of this shell, a shell so foreign and cumbrous that I found myself bumping into door frames, lamp shades, easy chairs. My size had come so quickly that I hadn't learned to accommodate it.

But by September of 1986, two years after I had first embraced iron, something went wrong. I ignored it at first. After all, the Medco was frequently unreliable. I upped my food dosages and supplements, but without effect. The cruel fact was my body had stuttered, then stopped growing. My training diary recorded the problem; the tape measure confirmed it. I was stuck with 17-inch arms, a 17-inch neck, 16-inch calves, a 48-inch chest, and 26-inch thighs. Months passed without a gain of even $\frac{1}{16}$ of an inch. In an agitated state, I confessed my problem to Sweepea.

He looked at me sympathetically, then bit his lip. "Plateau," he mumbled.

It is the word bodybuilders fear most. Somehow, some way, I had to break through it.

From what I could glean from the magazines, real builders, like Arnold, Bill Pearl, Lou Ferrigno—all of them had 20-inch necks, calves, and arms; 30-inch thighs; 60-inch chests. I was somewhere and nowhere at the same time. My muskets might have been the biggest in the Y, but they were nothing compared to the Gatling guns of bodybuilders from Southern California.

The "before" and "after" pictures of these bodybuilders were astounding. As soon as they reached sunny Southern California, their bodies seemed to explode in growth. The place had something: truckloads of anabolic steroids, variant exercise techniques, special diets—something. Whatever it was, if it worked for others, it might work for me. To the diseased there is only one Mecca, and it is nowhere near the nation of Islam.

My friends at the gym were delighted with my decision. They agreed: I was a bodybuilder, so I should move to Southern California. They were certain it would lead to layouts in the magazines. Only The Counter saved his words for himself, keeping up his recitation full-volume in the shower, as always.

I summoned my mother to meet me at the bunker to discuss the logistics of the move. The visit was a first for her. I heard her frightened tap at the first storm door. "Sam?" she squeaked.

She barely recognized me, but looked aghast at my uniform: military fatigues camouflaged to look like tree bark, spit-shined black combat boots, a T-shirt which read "Respect my spirit, for our spirits are one."

"Do we have bodybuilding to thank for this?" she asked bitterly.

"It's more than simply cosmetic, Mother," I said with gravity, "it's a whole way of life."

I swept my hand across the room. She took in the two ceiling-high refrigerators, the shelves of muscle magazines, the seated calf machine by my bed, and the smell of rotting food in the kitchenette. A cardboard cutout of Arnold with loincloth and sword as Conan the Barbarian stood against one wall. Sweepea had appropriated it from the marquee of a movie theater for me. Against another wall olive drab field utility boxes housed my protein powders, vitamins, and aminos. I could see from the look in her eyes that her worst fears were realized. All that was missing was a rifle and the President's travel itinerary.

She made her way to the bed and collapsed. "I'm sorry," she

said through her tears. "God, I'm so sorry." She clutched the iron-callused pads of my paw.

"That's all right, Mother," I heard myself saying, and, before I could stop myself, "no pain, no gain."

At this, the dam broke. She cried nonstop for a good ten minutes. And while I dabbed at her cheek with her handkerchief, I counted down the minutes until my next workout, and after that my westward flight.

I had done my job well. My own mother was crying on my breast and I didn't feel a thing. There wasn't a chink in my armor.

"A fresh start," I lied. "California. Clean air, a stable environment. It will all be good for me."

She looked up at me in misery. "To pursue this . . . this . . . bodybuilding thing?"

"Yes."

"But why?"

I gave her the standard party line. "It's an ambition to create something out of yourself that isn't there to start with, Mother. Like a sculptor, you play with the form and stretch it. I just want to see how far I can go."

That sounded nice, almost sane, in fact, but that wasn't what it was about at all, at least not for me. The fact was I'd found shelter in a body too large to feel and aimed to find even more in a body that was even bigger. It didn't occur to me then that too big might not be big enough.

"But where will this all end?" my mother asked.

"Lifting is a lifelong pursuit," I said with a smile, aping an article verbatim from the magazine open on my bed. "As long as I breathe, I lift. Without it . . ." again, the pause . . . "I shrivel up and die." I held out my palm and slowly balled it into a fist to emphasize the point.

More tears, but in the end she agreed to store my cartons of books beneath her desk in her apartment. *Muscle Wars*, *The Education of a Bodybuilder*, and *The Encyclopedia of Bodybuilding*, I took along with me. The clothes I gave to the Salvation Army. They no longer fit.

6.

THE MOVE

---

*WHATEVER IT IS YOU DO IN LIFE, YOU CAN
NEVER GROW IN SELF-ESTEEM UNLESS YOU GET
GOOD AND PUMPED FIRST AND STAY THAT WAY.
ANY TIME YOU SPEND WITHOUT A PUMP IS TIME
YOU CAN NEVER GET BACK AGAIN. I WOULDN'T
LET ANY OPPORTUNITIES GET AWAY IF I WERE
YOU.*

—FRANCO COLUMBU

O

ctober, 1986. In one hand, I held a large suitcase, in the other a Gold's Gym bag. The weight-lifting belt I wore around my waist, loosely buckled like a gunbelt. The amino Chewables, I popped into my mouth every few minutes. My pants were carefully cut off at each knee for maximum calf display. I had $12,000 in my pocket in traveler's checks, all that remained of my inheritance from my grandfather.

"Shangri-La Fitness Training Center," the flag said in gold letters, flapping above the gym's door in the breeze. The street was deserted, save for a beat-up 1971 Ford Maverick parked across from the gym. The black vinyl roof of the Maverick had blistered and peeled from the sun. The woven mat before the entrance didn't say "Welcome." It said, "Don't talk about it, do it!" The words were framed within a pattern of little dumbbells.

This was it. Southern California. Iron Mecca. Land of heavy artillery and for me, I hoped, opportunity. I took a deep breath and struggled with my bags through the door. The place was nearly empty. The DJ on the radio interrupted the rock music to announce "Your suntan turnover time is now three fifteen." To the left was a long, spotless counter; to the right a juice bar for protein shakes and other liquid power blasters. I stepped forward and held on to the gleaming, chrome gate and turnstile that fenced off the reception room from the free-weight area.

The weight room before me was huge—as large, in fact, as the Y's was small. Once a munitions factory, now a gym occupying 100,000 feet, it had at least two of everything: squat racks, Smith machines, bench presses, incline presses, and row after row of black iron dumbbells. You can always tell a serious gym by its heaviest dumbbells. A good gym will have a matching set that weigh 125 pounds each. A great one houses two monsters at 180 pounds apiece. I examined the dumbbell rack in the distance, and found what I was looking for. The 180-pounders sagged on the stand—just a foot and a half long, but as heavy as a large human being.

I couldn't imagine anyone strong enough to actually hoist these, until I heard the screams by the squat rack. There lumbered a mountain of a man squatting with 585 pounds on the bar. He stood as close to seven feet as six, and had shaved his white skull bald except for a thin arrow of black hair that started at the base of his medulla oblongata and ended an inch above his eyebrows. He had huge lips and no forehead. He wore a sweat-stained gray XXXL sweatshirt with L. Clement stenciled in black on the back.

"Like a human piston, Lamar! Like a human piston!" an older man with a white towel around his neck shouted behind him as Lamar performed his reps with harsh grunts and wild snorts. This rotund training partner wore an identical sweatshirt, stenciled with his own name, M. Clement. My own shirt was a parting gift from Sweepea and Mousie back at the Y. It depicted Fred Flintstone and Barnie Rubble "pumping granite" in a prehistoric weight room.

But Lamar and his partner weren't the only gym rats laboring on the floor. In every corner I saw them, "standing relaxed" like statues, and they were all at least twice my size. A man working on the dip bar was black and bald, like Mousie, but there the similarity ended. While Mousie had legs, and nothing else, he had everything. His arms alone had to measure over 20 inches, and they were covered with as many veins and bulges as a topographical roadmap.

And over by the preacher bench I saw, at last, a woman body-builder. Her body was covered with muscles, her face with makeup, which was running from her sweat. In a voice deeper than Paul Robeson's, she shouted "Fuckin' A!" at every bicep rep. What appeared to be the beginning of a beard descended like Spanish moss from her upper lip down to her chin. Her back brought to mind a mohair sweater. She wasn't quite a woman and she wasn't quite a man, but she was, unmistakably, a builder.

I heard a giggle, and a singsong voice from behind the counter. "Hi, it's a great day at Shangri-La Fitness Training Center! My name is Tara? And how can I do you?" she smiled, revealing a perfect, gleaming set of teeth.

She could not have been more than twenty, with bright green eyes and sun-streaked, teased blond hair which she wore in a ponytail. A shiny rubber tank top barely contained her sharply conical breasts. I marveled at the defiance of gravity and attributed it to progressive weight resistance training. I later learned it was surgery. With a quick wave of her hand, she motioned me over, as if she were going to tell me a secret.

"Hi, guy!" she shouted. "We'd love to squeeze you in for a full year, so long as you, the client, find that to your, like, satisfaction, you know? But, hey, you know, we have, like, one day plans, one week plans, ten day plans, one month plans, three month plans, and more, uh . . ." she paused, looking confused. "And who do I have the pleasure of addressing?" She cocked her head to the side and played with her hair with a nervous hand.

I did "the Walk" over to her slowly and deliberately. Keeping my lats flexed, I introduced myself. As soon as she shook my hand, she reeled back and shrieked.

"My gawd! The calluses! Is your moon, like, in retrograde or what?" Mouth open, she examined my palm.

"Really, guy, be straight with me. Are you, like, an immigrant laborer?" she asked.

"No, I'm a builder," I explained, nervously. Back in New York, I had been sure. But here, next to Lamar, the bald, black man, and the enormous she-beast, I wasn't so sure.

Tara kept hold of my hand, leaning forward over the counter, and said, so close I could smell her Bazooka bubble gum, "You know, Sam, like, I think your name is really rad! And you know what else? I have a feeling you'll like it here, like, totally. And I mean, from your hand alone, I can see you're a bodybuilder, and you know what they say about men with big hands, don't you?"

I looked at her warily.

"Come on, silly! Men with big hands wear big gloves!" She tilted her head back and laughed. Then, abruptly, her expression changed and she began her sales pitch.

"Now, I mean, did you know that all the big boys from the area come here? I mean, like, they all do. You've heard of Moses, right?" She pointed at the black behemoth I'd seen by the dip bar. "He won his weight class at the Fresno Classic last year, and placed second at Mr. Channel Islands. We have him. And, Vinnie, well," Tara thought for a moment, "he got first, I think, at Mr. North-eastern Greenwich two years ago."

Keeping her hand on mine, Tara looked deep into my eyes and whispered, "He's just *so* totally fine! I look at Vinnie and I think, like, anytime, buddy, just a-n-y-t-i-m-e! But that's between you, me, and the fencepost, right, Sam?

"And, oh, like, I almost forgot," she continued, cupping her mouth with her hand. "There's Raoul, the boss. He, like, runs the place, you know? He's won the Teenage Cal, the Cal, the America, the Universe. Raoul's done it all, and then some. See, Babe," Tara said smiling, "you can't help but get amped here just walking through the door! Now, I look at you, Sam, and what do I see? I see, like, a big guy who can go all the way. We provide the gym, you provide the sweat. I mean bods are definitely our business. Now, Sam, do you want to pay by cash, check, traveler's check, MasterCard, AmEx, or auto debit?" She whipped out the metal credit-card appliance from behind the counter.

Accompanied by the stereo sounds of Lamar screaming by the squat rack and Moses moaning by the dip bar, I swallowed hard, pulled out my traveler's checks, and paid $400.00 for the full year.

"Whoa! I mean, like, to the max! That shirt is just *so* totally rad. I mean, like, where'd you get it?" Another blond, teased thing, with a nose as curved as a ski jump, came up behind me. She wore a rubberized, glossy tube top like Tara's, black tights, and a black lace G-string over them. She shuffled energetically to join Tara behind the counter, taking tiny geisha steps, since she hadn't quite mastered her 6-inch, spiked heels.

She stuck out a hand decorated with impossibly long, curved, pink nails but quickly withdrew it when I put my hand out to meet hers.

"Sorry, like, no offense or anything," she giggled, waving her fingers in front of her chest. "It's just that one of them broke again, so, you know, like, bummer, I had to put it back on, and then, you know, why not paint the whole set again? *My* name is Xandra and *my* motto is 'let's party?' And you are—?"

"That's Sam," Tara said, pointing her finger at me. "He's a body-builder and a new male member."

"Oh you *are?*" Xandra asked. "I'm *so* stoked! I mean, you're definitely buff, and you can tell just *so* much about a person by their body. I hate fat people, like, to the *max*, don't you? I mean they're just *so* lazy and things. Like, if you don't have respect for your body, guy, then what *do* you have? Like, whenever I pass some load, I don't know whether to stick a finger down *my* throat or *theirs*," she said, steadying a pocket mirror and calmly plucking at an eye-brow.

Health fascists and gym bunnies—it was my introduction to the major-league bodybuilding scene. And as soon as Tara and Xandra buzzed me through the chrome turnstile, I espied the rest of them. There seemed to be a California uniform code in effect. The men wore their standard issue: pastel-colored genie pants (oversize cotton bloomers with drawstrings at the waist and at each ankle), oversized Gold's Gym sweatshirts (carefully ripped at the neck to expose the trapezius muscles), Gold's Gym baseball caps decorated with small buttons (one said "Pray for War," another "I'd rather be killing Communists in Central America").

And as the men were dressed for building, the women were dressed for breeding. All of them favored the colorful, clinging tights, G-strings, tube tops, and other lingerie items modeled by Tara and Xandra. All of them, save G-spot, given name Dot, that is. She was the hirsute female builder I'd seen earlier whose construction boots, fatigues, and olive drab tank top signaled the Army/Navy store rather than Frederick's of Hollywood.

One fashion accessory indispensable to both sexes was the heavy leather weight-lifting belt. It was available in the pro shop in sturdy brown or black leather or multicolored suede. Some lifters carried them over their shoulders like bandoliers, others buckled them so tightly around their waists that it looked like their upper bodies would pop from the pressure. The biggest men, though—Lamar and Moses included—wore theirs loosely, like a carpenter's utility belt, between sets. The belts, for the most part, were unnecessary in the gym, only needed for back support for a few exercises. But they were vital for purposes of collective identity, which is why they were worn at all times. I'd worn mine on the plane ride out.

It certainly was different from what I had expected. My only previous experience with California gyms were the ones I had seen in the backgrounds of the muscle magazines. I had spent hundreds of hours back in the bunker hovering over these photographs, a bottle of rubber cement on my desk, pasting my head on different bodies. The gyms in these shots were cold, Spartan, undecorated, the kind where none of the lifters wore shirts, but most of them wore tattoos, the kind where you would expect to find a sign by the front door saying: "No rugs, no sauna, just iron."

But Shangri-La looked like a cross between a cathedral and a singles bar. Every corner housed a fern. A series of Casablanca fans hummed from the 20-foot ceiling. Skylights in the roof created spotlights on the floor, illuminating iron worshipers in a fountain of fiery brilliance. Between the lifters, a score of neatly clad, pencil-necked employees in red uniforms officiously replaced the weights in the racks and cleaned the equipment. There were framed, signed photographs of bodybuilders and airbrushed lithographs of stream-lined nudes by Patrick Nagel on the redbrick walls.

The dominating decorations of the gym, though, were a series of life-size blown-up photographs of the owner, Raoul, posing in his competition briefs. There were twenty of these, all black-and-white, slung from the wooden rafters like flags in a medieval banquet hall. He was the equal to just about anyone I'd seen in the magazines. I knew that to get that spectacular a body would take me at least six more years of three on, one off, double-split sessions, forced feeding combined with stringent dieting, and, of course, complete focus. At the very least, six years. It might well take thirty-five or forty years, as it had for the bodybuilder Albert Beckles, now still competing at the age of sixty.

But I didn't stop for even a moment to consider the effort or, for that matter, the absurdity of the quest. Instead, displaying again the symptoms of the diseased, I rushed off to the locker room to pursue my career choice by shaving a few nubs off my legs with my Lady Bic. While I was exchanging the tank top I wore on the street for the one I wore in the gym, I saw a near-naked figure at the mirror.

"Seven percent," he said smugly.

He was "standing relaxed" in his underwear, with his shirt in one hand and his pants rolled down around his ankles.

He turned his head to me. "I'm seven percent," he said again. "Body fat," he added, proffering his hand.

With his free hand, he dug his fingers into my side, using his thumb and index finger as makeshift calipers. "You're about twelve percent," he said grimacing, "probably even more."

There was something about his face—he looked familiar. Suddenly it hit me. The posters outside. This was Raoul, Mr. America.

"You . . . you . . . you look so different," I stammered.

Raoul smiled, revealing a latticework of metal in his mouth. "It's the braces," he said firmly. But it wasn't the braces. It was the body. In the pictures, he looked enormous, a Master of the Universe. In person, he looked like a malnourished accountant.

Raoul saw the look of confusion on my face. "I know what you're thinking," he said. "I'm a little old for braces. Well, maybe, but it's a marketing decision. It will help my overall presentation."

I nodded my head and donned my sneakers. Raoul, glimpsing himself in the mirror again, couldn't contain his excitement. "Hey buddy, look and learn," he said. "Watch me expose my rectus abdominus!"

He shifted on his feet, offered his right side to the mirror, and, in a deliberate motion, lifted his right arm above his head before tilting his right hip in the direction of the mirror. He nodded rigorously at the sight. His abdominal muscles looked like an ice-cube tray. He had but one more word to say, "Quality." With a little smirk, he pulled his clothes back on and strutted out the door.

As soon as he left, I tried the move myself. The rectus abdominus was nowhere to be found. My body-fat percentage was simply too high. Where Raoul had a deeply gouged grid of rectangular brown muscles, I had a pasty blanket of white flesh.

I might have despaired had I not heard the thundering steps of Lamar behind me. His wild dash didn't stop until he had emptied his guts into the toilet right by my posing mirror.

"Lamar! Son!" his father (and training partner) cried, waving a towel before him, as he rushed in a few seconds afterwards. The old man fell to his knees to cradle his son's head in his arms, then helped his massive offspring right himself from the messy bowl.

My response was automatic and a little too loud. "The muscles gained are worth the price of the pain," I said, covering my love handles with my tank top and the iron shibboleth.

Lamar's father broke into a grin at my words and introduced himself.

"I'm Lamar's dad, Macon's the name." He was the first person I'd seen who didn't look like he modeled for *Muscle Digest* or *Penthouse*. "Say, weren't you in the heavies last year at Mr. Ironman?" Macon asked, biting his fingernails and knitting his brow in an effort to remember.

"No, I'm filling out before I compete. I'll compete in a city show next year," I revealed. I knew that much; start off with a city show, take it to the state, then the nationals. . . .

Lamar peeked out from his stall and came to join us. His father carefully swabbed the corners of his mouth, as Lamar held both hands to his head and moaned in pain.

"Lamar, we got us a new builder," Macon said.

Lamar looked up and brightened visibly. When he discovered I was from New York, like his idol Lou Ferrigno, he asked me all about the legendary New York gyms, like Tom Minichiello's Mid-City in Manhattan, and Julie Levine's R & J in Brooklyn. I'd heard of both but hadn't dared to work out at either. I admitted no such thing, though, instead trumpeting my workouts in them and the good times I'd shared with the owners.

Suddenly, Lamar looked at himself in the mirror in a panic. He turned to Macon and said: "Oh no, Dad, look! Oh no! I've lost some size!" They both glanced back at the toilet in misery.

I dashed to my locker and brought back a pack of BIG Chewables. As luck would have it, Lamar and I used the same brand, and he popped a handful of these into his mouth, along with a multivitamin pack I gave him, as though they were candy. The effect on Lamar was immediate. He did "the Walk" all over the locker room.

Thanking me for my generous care for a fellow builder, Macon asked if I would be so kind as to join him and the elephantine Lamar after the workout at their Ford Maverick, which was parked across the street. They called the Maverick home, Macon confided. He was going to barbecue some chicken and vegetables, laced with protein powder—only bodybuilding foods, he assured me. I promised I would join them as soon as I finished my own workout.

It was while I was on the seated calf machine that day that I first heard the ruckus. My head was down, my face contorted in agony. I'd been at it for a full hour, painfully isolating my soleus and gastrocnemius muscles. To really "get into" them, I was, of course, using the usual visualization procedure, in this case seeing my calves as gigantic spinnakers close to bursting from the force of a raging sea squall. My concentration was broken by the roar of a deep voice.

"In the final arena, there will be no judges, only witnesses to my greatness!" proclaimed an immense figure in a New York accent, hopping over the turnstile at the front door. He proceeded to do "the Walk" over to the squat platform. And oh what a walk he did! I had never seen quads thrust so far apart in the eternal battle against chafing, or arms suspended at such a distance from the body. And the majestic motion—so slow it took him a good 45 seconds to travel 30 feet.

He wore a silk do-rag over his head, a kind of colorful kerchief popular among minority women and gang members in depressed urban pockets of the United States. Over his massive and heavily acned torso, he sported a Gold's Gym tank top and sweatshirt. The sweatshirt was ripped just enough around the collar to reveal a jutting and greasy pair of trapezius muscles. On his legs he wore, direct from Marrakesh, billowing genie pants the color of orange sherbert. The outfit was completed by purple socks and black Reeboks.

"Oh yes!" he screamed at the top of his lungs, nodding his head up and down dramatically. "Oh yes, we have come to train today! May we say it?" Without waiting for an answer, he burst forth with "Yes, I think we may. This is *serious* business!" Most of the other lifters, especially the smaller ones, gave him wide clearance.

"Do the right thing, buddy, do the right thing!" the hulk bellowed to himself. He shook his head from side to side, revealing the feathered earring that reached down to tickle one of his traps. Tightening his belt and wrist straps, he strode to the mirror to arrange his do-rag. He lingered for a moment at the mirror before rushing to the deadlift bar to warm up with 225 pounds for 15 lighting-quick reps. On his last rep, with a great clatter, he threw the bar from him in disgust, and did "the Walk" to the water fountain. There he lollygagged to slowly lick his flexed bicep for Tara and Xandra.

Xandra shrieked and hid under the counter. Tara, bolt upright, mouth slightly open, hips pressed forward against the counter's edge, didn't take her eyes off him.

On his way back to the platform, the hulk caught a smaller man eyeing him with distaste. Walking right up to him, he sneered, "Yeah? Don't break your pencil case, geek. Why don't you go get Raoul, huh? I spit on the both of you, you little closet shits!"

The target of his vehemence turned completely red, and fled in fear to the locker room. Clearly, it made the hulk's day. His heavily muscled arm was raised in triumph; he flourished his clenched fist. He did "the Walk" back to the squat platform, where for ten brutal repetitions he deadlifted 405 pounds.

"Make haste slowly," I reminded myself, resisting the urge to run over and join him. His act was familiar to me. It reminded me of the free-weight section back at the Y. But it was clear that it didn't go over well in this California gym.

No wonder. Back in New York, lifting had been about war. Here, judging from the conversations around me, it was about net-working. The hard-core builders were there, true; the Axles, the Bulldozers, the Guses (the usual nerds were in attendance as well— the Norberts and Nestors). But they were all swamped by the crowd of Kips and Corkys and Alistaires who flooded through the door after five o'clock. And that went for the women, too. The Ramonas, Desirées, and Dulcies were now few; the Catherines, and Jennifers, and Victorias many. Back at the Y, "opportunities for advancement" had meant the squat rack and the bench press. Here, it seemed to mean vocational choices and personal investments. The air was heavy with speculation on the vagaries of CDs, IRAs, and prime rates.

The one throwback to an earlier era was this blustering bully. As I watched, he skipped from the water fountain to the deadlifting bar. He sang the following ditty at the top of his lungs, while he chalked his palms and fingers and adjusted his wrist straps in preparation for the lift:

> One, two, three, four,
> Every night I pray for war!
> Five, six, seven, eight,
> Rape, kill, mutilate!

As if it were nothing, he picked up the 500 pounds on the deadlift bar and brought it up to his hips, repeating the movement for 10 strict reps. I was amazed. His face bore a rapt expression, as if nothing could please him more than being here and doing this. When I did it, for one pathetic rep, my whole body shuddered from the pain.

"We're talkin' big man muscles, goddamnit, I mean, serious muscles, I mean, we're talkin' *big!*" he yelled at the mirror again, his straining, screaming face one inch from the glass. His face and upper back bore the deep pits and craters of endless acne bombardments. His bulging traps were decorated with gigantic boils and cysts. He looked as happy as a pig in slop.

The workout as operatic drama, with all the peaks and sloughs known to each. In body and performance, he was light-years beyond Sweepea and Mousie. Here was joy. Here was fierceness.

I couldn't restrain myself a second longer. I did "the Walk" over to the dumbbell rack, and imitated the master. As a sign of the extraordinary purity of my own muscle isolation, I wailed like a banshee through my reps to the astonished stares of even the biggest builders present. My shrieks simply recapitulated a gloss from the book *Pumping Iron*. Gaines and Butler observed Arnold during his workouts and noticed that he made a great deal more noise than his training partners during his exercises. They attributed it to the essential purity of Arnold's lifting movements. Since his form was impeccable, his horrible cries and tortured looks were the result of really knowing how to isolate and exercise the muscles without resorting to the cowardice of cheating. The magazines called this

"Muscle Integrity." Accompanied by the sonic booms of the hulk's deadlifting, I sang a little melody of my own while I did my arm curls.

"I saw a bird on the window sill," I screamed, pausing in my lyrics until I had completed a 60-pound dumbbell rep with one arm.

"Singin' fine and sittin' still," I continued, doing another rep, this time with the other arm.

"I coaxed him in with a piece of bread!" Another rep.

"Then I crushed his little head!" I sang, fortissimo, completing verse and set. A feeling of contentment spread through my body; I was at peace with myself, my pump, world.

The hulk had heard me singing from his side of the room. He came striding over, his do-rag flowing in the wind.

"Hey, uh, yo, like uh, you from England or somethin'?" he asked, tilting his head and hiking up his pants.

"No, New York," I said. It sounded more prudent than Princeton.

As soon as the words passed my lips, the hulk clutched me to his breast in friendship, repeating over and over again, the words "Semper Fi, Mac, Semper Fi."

Of such moments are bonds made. On my very first day, I had found a training partner, and his name was Vinnie. As soon as he released me, he hiked up his pants again. Looking down, I saw beneath his weight-lifting belt what appeared to be a white plastic retaining liner partially hidden beneath the fabric of his genie pants.

It didn't click then, but it should have. The hulk was wearing Huggies, the superabsorbent diaper built to contain any accident, no matter how extreme. I later learned that during the rigors of his deadlifting sessions, Vinnie had need of several per workout (he fastened two pairs together with, yes, safety pins). Thus equipped, he could concentrate solely on the lift at hand. No embarrassment, no failure. His record was a full box for one session—one record I didn't want to break.

That afternoon, leaving the gym together, we vowed to meet for legs the next morning. Vinnie had eschewed a shower, since he believed it made him lose weight. I did the same, willing to try anything to break my plateau.

I gave him the soul shake by the door and, remembering Macon and Lamar's offer of hospitality, struggled with my bags to the Maverick. In turn, Vinnie climbed up into his Chevy Luv pickup truck, which he had customized with a lift kit, sixteen raised shock absorbers and giant tires. The body of the car was so high off the ground it looked like something out of Dr. Seuss. He raised his hand and gave me a wave as he put it in gear.

"How do you like my wheels?" Vinnie shouted, above the roar of the engine.

"Hot, it's hot!" I said.

Vinnie looked at me startled. "How did you know?"

As I was to learn, Vinnie's truck was, in fact, stolen. Or rather, parts of it were. He had a Toyota hood, Ford doors, and a GMC engine. The vehicle was a "chop-shop special."

When he saw me heading in the direction of the Maverick, he screeched his monstrous amalgam to a halt. "Hey, Sam, are you residin' uh, chez Macon and Lamar this evenin'?"

I nodded.

"I'll see what I can cook up fo' you, New York," he said, putting his car back in gear, a determined glint in his eye. I watched the Chevy roar down the street. There was a vanity license plate on the back. In bold letters, it said: POWER. Around it, Vinnie had attached a chrome frame, which read "You be the six, I'll be the nine."

"Come on over, Sam. Take a load off!" I heard Macon's voice from behind the Maverick. He opened the truck and stuffed my bags in. Among the gym attire, the straps, the belts, the arm blasters and neck harnesses, there was very little room. Lamar shyly shook my hand and introduced me to his pit bull Cuddles, who bared his fangs in greeting.

We retired to the lawn chairs Macon had set up on the sidewalk by the barbecue, a few feet from the Maverick. Macon rose to offer me a full plate full of hot chicken breasts, some vegetables, and a container of nonfat milk mixed with high-grade protein powder and carbohydrate concentrate. I took the plate, thanked them kindly, and settled into the chair Lamar gently slid my way.

As I eased into the lawn chair, Macon spoke of his hopes and physique aspirations for his son. Lamar was eating well, he said, his lifts were in order, his supplementation was of a consistently high dosage. Macon had even purchased Cuddles for him, since he had read in a physique monthly that pets reduce stress (and stress, of course, causes mental and physical depletion).

While I listened to Macon, I set about ripping the trapezius sections out of all of my new Gold's Gym sweatshirts with the aid of my commando knife. He was still talking as we cooled down with the protein coladas Lamar made with the blender.

"Do you think bodybuilding is in a healthy phase right now, Sam?" Macon asked, testing me while he bit into a carob power-explosion bar.

"How do you mean?" I asked, chewing a desiccated beef-liver tablet.

"Let me put it to you this way, son. Who is your favorite body-builder?"

"No contest," I said. "Arnold."

Lamar and his father exchanged delighted glances.

"And after him, Sam, who do you think you'd like to be?"

I thought to myself, this time for a good fifteen silent seconds. No one else came to mind, myself least of all.

"Arnold," I said again.

"Right on, Sam!" Macon cried, slapping his hand against his knee. "See, goshdarn it, that's just what I mean! Now, you look at these shrunken poodles that pass for Mr. Universe these days," he said, showing me a well-thumbed magazine with a particularly emaciated specimen in green posing trunks on its cover. Lamar smiled and nodded his head vigorously from his chair. I knew the builder and the magazine. I had a subscription. "For God's sake," Macon said, exasperated, "I'll tell you somethin': You jus' give me one of them starvin' Biafrans, and I'll show you muscle striations. I mean have you seen the abs and intercostals on some of them guys? But my God, how come human ropes like, like . . . Raoul are tryin' to pass themselves off as lifters, I ask you?

"Now dagnabit, Sam, it don't take no genius to know that Lamar ain't never gonna pass for one of them clipped poodles, but, in God's name, why the hell (pardon my French, Lamar) should he?

"I mean, take one look at the man. He's paid his dues! Doggone it, he's a Clydesdale in a world of Shetland ponies!" Macon spat out a chicken bone to emphasize the point.

Looking over at Lamar, I saw a thirty-year-old, 325-pound man with an arrowhead haircut pretending to read a magazine called *Four Wheeler*. I say pretending, because he was rocking in his chair, holding Cuddles to him with all his might, basking in his father's approbation.

Macon pointed a long, loving finger at his son. "That's it in a nutshell, Sam," he said. "I mean, strike me blind if Lamar's off-season weight ain't a biscuit away from 350, if he's a pound! It just ain't healthy these days. It's like you got to carry 'round one a them diuretics manuals just to take to the posin' dais!

"I mean you can have your Mohamed Makkawys, your Samir Bannouts, your Pierre Vandensteens," Macon said, with a dismissive wave of his hand at foreign builders in general. "Pile 'em all together on the Medco, and they still don't add up to one Lamar!"

Lamar smiled at his father, and slowly rose from his chair. So far he hadn't said a word. He trusted Macon with Cuddles and grabbed two more chicken breasts from the barbecue.

Back in his seat, Lamar spoke in a slow, sorrowful tone. "I have faith, Sam, strong faith," he said. "And you know, I see things this way: Since the beginning of time, human beings have crucified our lord Jesus Christ and plagued the land with all kinds of pestilences and wars. Now, if people can do that to whole civilizations through the course of time, then just imagine the world of hurt they can put on me, unless I watch my six. I put my trust in no one, no one but Cuddles, Dad, and heavy lifters. Heavy lifters like you, Sam. My motto is 'If you hear me growlin', man, don't come rattle my cage.' "

"Now, now, Lamar, don't get all agitated," Macon said. "Don't you remember what I told you 'bout stress? Here, quick, take Cuddles."

Lamar nodded silently, and retreated to his lawn chair.

"Anyway," Macon continued. "It's just like I told you yesterday, son, these things go in cycles. All you got to do is open a book and examine history. Now, son, the late sixties and early seventies were a time when size ruled, with them Arnolds and Sergio Olivas and Lou Ferrignos. Then—kind of like what the good book says—

a darkness fell over the land, 'cause the mid-seventies came and those Frank Zanes and sunken-cheeked foreigners ruled the stage. I mean, why would anybody in their right mind pay to see some guy with a Chippendale's physique? But now, thanks to Lee Haney, we might be coming back to good times, Arnold times, Lamar times."

"I'd rather be Bertil Fox and never win an Olympia, than be Frank Zane, and win three," Lamar recited by rote, clutching Cuddles to him. I recognized the names. They represented two physique extremes: Bertil Fox looked like a refrigerator with veins, Frank Zane like a prisoner of war. Each had been popular in his day.

That first starry California night I spent with Lamar, Macon, and Cuddles in the Maverick. Lamar retired with Cuddles to the back seat. Macon took the passenger side, and I made the best of it with the wheel and the pedals of the driver's side.

From my vantage point behind the wheel, I stared at the air freshener which hung from the rear view mirror. It smelled like a Vermont forest, but it was shaped like a dumbbell. On it were the words: "Bodybuilders do it . . . until it hurts."

Amid the silence, I heard Lamar stir in the back seat. Making sure his father was asleep, he pressed forward and rested a hand the size of a catcher's mitt on my shoulder. A confession was coming up, I could feel it. I braced myself for the worst. What would it be? Homicide, genocide, or, casting a glance at Macon snoozing beside me, patricide?

"Sam," Lamar whispered in his doomsday voice. "I think of myself as a chocolate popsicle in creation. You know, at first in the factory, you just have the popsicle stick. That's like, the way we were born, what the good Lord gave us. Then, you dip the stick into a hotbed of chocolate, and you get a coating. See, more coatings mean more muscles. The gym is the hotbed of chocolate, Sam, and we're the popsicles. After ten or fifteen years of repeated applications, you got yourself one humongous chocolate popsicle."

"Lamar," I said, relieved, "you're a natural born poet."

"Ain't every bodybuilder?" Lamar asked, settling into comfort with Cuddles.

"Right on, Lamar!" Macon shouted, a tear falling from his eye. He hadn't been asleep after all.

I loosened my weight-lifting belt, slumped back in my seat, and tried to get some sleep. Shangri-La, Open 24 Hours, was our night-light that evening, and Macon and Lamar fell fast asleep to the lullaby of iron clinking across the street. Mercifully, I slipped into unconsciousness soon after.

7.

THE JUICE

IN THE QUEST FOR THAT WINNING EDGE, THE ADVANTAGE OVER ONE'S OPPONENT, MANY ATHLETES HAVE OPTED TO DIG DEEPER INTO THEIR PHARMACEUTICAL GRAB-BAG.

—*FRED HATFIELD*

The next morning, I waited at the juice bar for Vinnie. We were to train legs at nine A.M. From my position on the stool by the counter, I sipped my Blueberry Force Primeval Shake and listened to the noises indigenous to the California gym.

Xandra, on the phone with a girlfriend, was shocked. "You're kidding!" she squealed. "My God, that's, like, such a coincidence! I can't believe Cerise! Did you know that I see *my* channeler once every two weeks too! Last time, she got these really neat tapes of Jock—that's my spiritual contact, you know—talking through *her* voice. I mean I'm so into that I just can't decide *what* I should pursue in the long run. Like, metaphysics, or hand modeling?" She stretched her nails, dry now, out before her.

From the weight room, I heard Macon forcing another rep out of Lamar on the bench press.

"Work it, son, work it!" Macon yelled. "Feel the hardness of it, watch it grow!"

Beside me, a beefy man lifted his head from his Strawberry Carbo Fuel Supreme Shake (with extra protein powder and nonfat yogurt) at the sound of his girlfriend at the door.

"Tony, I'm going to the salon, do you want me to pick you up some gel?" she queried. She brushed a spritz-soaked lock of hair from her eyes, and adjusted her halter top.

Tony grunted his response. His calves had the girth of my thigh. Arnold, in his *Encyclopedia*, mentioned that calves like those cost at least 500 hours of straining, tortuous calf sessions. "Great calves," I said in admiration. "You must have paid a heavy price."

"You got that right," Tony said, flexing them for our mutual benefit. "3,500 bucks. Implants. Dr. Rebus over in Woodland Hills did them. You've heard of him, right?—he does a lot of builders. He just inserts a little sheath in each, and presto, instant calves." He looked down at my legs. "I'll give you his card," he said in sympathy, and then whispered mysteriously, "He can cut out your gyno, too," before heading off for his workout.

There I sat, dressed in my new genie pants, Reeboks, oversized Gold's Gym sweatshirt and cap, mentally preparing for the onslaught of Vinnie's arrival. It was different from New York, but not that different. Minutes earlier I had suffered another painful bout of diarrhea. This time it wasn't skells or the urban inferno, it was legs with Vinnie. I feared I might not be able to hang with him, as they say in the gym, matching him pound for pound, exercise for exercise.

Macon had told me over breakfast that Vinnie believed in "intensity or insanity," a training method popularized by Vinnie's mentor, the onetime Mr. America, Steve Michalik. Most bodybuilders adhere to the theory that four or five exercises per body part, with four or five sets per exercise, is more than enough for any one workout, and that anything more than twenty-five total sets per 90 minutes or two hours is overtraining. But not Michalik or his disciples. They often did as many as fifty sets per body part, using a full two hours just to train one muscle. This necessitated a few adjustments, using less weight and more reps, for instance, with little rest between sets. It also involved a muscle principle known as "continuous tension," in which the builder shortens his range of motion from four-fourths of a movement to three-fourths. By eliminating the pause at the top of the movement (that last fourth), the lifter ensures that the muscles are constantly, continually at work.

From what I gathered from Macon, Vinnie alternated his training style, some days bombing his muscles with this "intensity or insanity," other days slowing down the workouts and permitting pauses, doing fewer sets and reps in the hope that the heavier weights he used would help him pack on more size. I knew that I would have to experience both methods if I were to break my plateau and continue growing, but I was apprehensive and, most of all, scared. After all, I didn't know which to prepare myself for: the blinding pace of high reps or the slow, deliberate, numbing pain of strength training.

At last, I heard the voice of my partner. "Oh yeah! Let's rock 'n' roll, Sam!" Vinnie screamed, as he strode in and spotted me at the juice bar.

"Two hundred forty-two pounds and hard!" Vinnie announced with his arms outspread, referring to his own muscular condition.

He pointed one hand in the direction of the squat rack and the other at me. "Sam, prepare to meet thy doom!" he shouted, throwing down the gauntlet.

Vinnie wore the same outfit as the day before; the only variant was the do-rag. I asked him about his clothes. He said he never washed them. The laundromat had nothing to do with the gym, so why waste the energy? I gave him a little fist salute of iron man solidarity, breathing through my mouth rather than my nose to keep from gagging at the stench.

That morning, when Vinnie took his knee wraps, his belt, and his ammonia capsules out of his Gold's Gym bag, I realized that it would not be an "intensity or insanity" day. It would be a strength day.

So began my education. Where Vinnie traveled, I followed. I couldn't help it—we were tethered to the same Sony Walkman Vinnie wore in a black leather fanny pack around his waist. The machine housed a port for two headsets at a time, and my cord let me wander no more than 10 feet.

Vinnie and I first did "I go/you-go." We started at the leg extension machine, 15 reps each. As soon as he finished his set, I hopped on; when I finished, he hopped on. The weights we used were abnormally light, just a warm-up before squats. My concentration was broken only by the sound of Vinnie's encouragement: "That's right, Big Man! Don't you let up! Goddamnit, rip that door right off its fuckin' hinges!"

He told me we would do about ten sets of squats. This was unusual. Few lifters exceed five, and for good reason. After the sixth set (and fifteenth repetition) I took off the headset, staggered outside and vomited the half-dozen raw eggs Macon had given me for breakfast and the protein shake Tara had made for me at the juice bar.

For a moment, I was ashamed. I felt I'd let down the side. As soon as I reentered the room, I attacked the weights with ferocity. It was the right thing to do. Get back on the horse and ride. Vinnie's admiration was unbounded. He was inspired.

"Like a freight train from hell, baby! Oh yes!" he screamed. "I got myself a real trainin' partner!"

From behind me, I heard Macon as well. "All day long, Sam!" he yelled. He told Vinnie that, in some ways, I reminded him of Lamar. We were dinosaurs, true, he said, but we weren't extinct yet.

Vinnie began to load up the squat rack with 400, then 500, then 600 pounds. I couldn't lift this successfully on my own; I wasn't strong enough. So with the bar bent over my back, Vinnie wrapped his arms around my waist and tugged me up from the floor at every rep. Forced squat reps. With 600 pounds. Even with my knees wrapped and my back secured with my belt, I couldn't believe the pain.

For his own set, Vinnie stopped communing with the other lifters. For him, the heavier weight necessitated a certain manner of preparation. He retreated to his own private world, reserved for all kinds of rituals, ceremonies, and ammonia capsules. He paced nervously around the squat bar for 90 long seconds. Then, a tightening of his weight belt, and a run over to my direction. He stopped a foot from me to point at his legs and scream: "Look at these fuckin' gams, Sam! These are manly gams, goddamnit!" He quickly flexed them in the mirror and caressed them with a loving hand, before snatching an ammonia capsule from my open palm. Breaking it directly under his nose, he inhaled deeply, looked as if he'd just seen God, then rushed to the squat bar, where he tightened his belt and settled in under it.

At this point, he rocked on his feet, head-butting the steel bar several times in an effort to initiate an adrenal spurt. Finally, with his mind focused from the ammonia and his forehead gushing blood, he performed the exercise.

On his heaviest set, 645 pounds even, he asked me, as his

training partner, to "do the right thing." From my acquaintance with
Powerlifting USA magazine, I realized what he meant. After his knee
wrap, his walk, his talk, his ammonia intake, and his belt ritual, I
nailed him twice with a closed fist and clean shots to the face. The
result was a bloody nose, a black eye, and a successful lift. In the
world outside the gym, they call it assault and battery. Inside the
gym and in the magazines, it's called the "Heightened Arousal Mode"
("making *your* anger work for *you!*"). It's what I'd seen Sweepea and
Mousie doing in amateur fashion that first night back at the Y.

But it wasn't all just sound and fury. Above the roar of his
Walkman, Vinnie taught me how to adjust the stance of my feet
on every leg exercise in order to change the shape of my quadriceps.
I learned to keep my ankles together, and my feet facing straight
forward to build up the outside sweep of my thigh (for the vastus
lateralis muscle). I learned to splay my feet in an open stance, like
a duck, to add muscular layers on to my "teardrop" muscle (known
as the vastus medialis) that in the biggest builders drapes over the
knee.

In fact, Vinnie had a positional variation, for every exercise and
body part, which made the gym, for an advanced builder like himself, a kind of mail-order catalog. Instead of money, Vinnie ex-
pended energy and outfitted his body with muscles of his own design
rather than clothes.

And I was a quick study. Vinnie had never seen a pupil like me.
I was the only training partner he'd ever had who barfed as a matter
of course. During workouts, the only face more contorted in pain
than his was mine. To my surprise, except for Macon and Lamar,
we were the only ones who seemed even to be trying.

The other men and women around us, the fashionably thin rather
than the fashionably muscular, did their exercises in an expression-
less trance. I asked Vinnie about this. Was it a new technique? A
special visualization process? Not at all, said Vinnie, the more you
scrunched up your face, the more lines you developed. These shop-
window mannequins were trying to preserve their faces, to protect
them from premature aging.

To Vinnie the whole matter was simple. "Shit, buddy, you don't
get to be no air stewardess lookin' like that!" he said, pointing at

G-spot. She grimaced and sneered while she worked her back. According to Vinnie, though she was barely twenty-three, she would soon bear the wrinkles of a beldam.

At the juice bar after the workout, Vinnie bought me a 2½-ounce jar of baby food. It was Gerber's Junior Meat Beef. At first, I thought him joking, but when I turned to Lamar I saw that he, too, was savoring a tiny something in his huge hands. You could barely see it, but there it was. Peach Cobbler, of the Gerber Junior Dessert series. All builders swore by them; they were great protein and carbohydrate sources. I suppressed a smile as Vinnie handed me a jar of Junior Chicken Noodle and a baby spoon.

It wasn't enough for Vinnie to feed me. Like Macon and Lamar the previous night, he offered me shelter. It was settled, he told me. He had already discussed the matter with his roommates, Nimrod and Bamm Bamm. If I wanted, I could stay with them. It wouldn't be an inconvenience—they had an extra room. Besides, as my behavior amply proved, I was family.

So it was I found myself using the chrome stirrup bolted to the cab and clambering unsteadily into Vinnie's customized, jacked-up, turbo-charged pickup. Vinnie had changed into his work clothes: tights and a loose Gold's Gym sweatshirt, with a Gold's Gym baseball cap he wore back-to-front on his balding crown. A small button was attached to his Gold's Gym baseball cap. It read Gold's Gym.

In a sense, I had truly struck gold with Vinnie. He was a bodybuilder's bodybuilder. When obstacles arose in his path, whether in the gym or on the street, he forcibly removed them. As he put it, blaring his horn, cutting off other motorists, pausing at stoplights to hector the cars beneath us, "Yeah, Sam, why jus' drive when you can rule the road? That's my motto, anyway."

On the mad dash to 1404 Delacey, Vinnie found time, between bouts of swearing at other drivers, to brief me on his two roommates, both bodybuilders. According to Vinnie, Nimrod had class, Bamm Bamm mass. I understood. Nimrod had cuts, or the chiseled look, Bamm Bamm size.

Vinnie parked the car in the middle of the front lawn of my new home. I smiled and waved at Nimrod and Bamm Bamm, waiting at the door. Neither of them spoke a word of greeting. Nimrod, like Vinnie, about five ten, had long blond hair that cascaded in a multiple series of tiny braids to his spinal erectors. Below the hair was the body. He was a human anatomy chart. His skin was as transparent as rice paper and beneath that gauze I saw a trellis of capillaries, veins, and arteries. His body fat was so freakishly low that every muscle fiber beneath the skin visibly shook and swayed with every movement.

Bamm Bamm was simply huge. So huge, in fact, that from a distance, his tiny head looked like a pea resting on a ruler. He was Lamar's size, but, my intuition told me, not quite so gentle. His clenched fists indicated that.

The place reminded me of The Growth Center back in New York. The floors were strewn with back issues of *Muscle & Fitness*, *Ironman*, *Flex*, as well as the lesser known *Ironsport*, *Muscular Development*, *Modern Bodybuilding* and *National Physique Committee News*. The living room was a messy tangle of chalk, stray lifting belts, wrist straps, knee wraps, spare ammonia capsules, used jocks, baby powder. The kitchen refrigerator was covered with dozens of cutout photographs of bodybuilding champions displaying their wares on the beach. Some beefy models posed outside tropical hotels, protein powder in one hand, a dazzling blonde in the other. Others were caught in the sweaty precincts of gyms, straining during a deadlift or a clean and press. One color shot showed a shirtless Lee Haney (the current Mr. Olympia, beloved by Macon and Lamar), spreading his lats, astride a smoking manhole cover clad only in blue jeans and black Reeboks. Another showed Anja Langer, an up-and-coming star from Germany, spreading her legs onstage, peeking seductively at the crowd from beneath a bronzed thigh.

But something was amiss. Though the familiar environment was reassuring, there was an unspoken hostility in the air. I'd felt it as soon as I'd walked through the door. It was Bamm Bamm and Nimrod. They had circled their wagons, still not proffering a word in my direction. Not when I unpacked my things in my new room, not when I put up a poster of Arnold on my new wall, not even when I added my tins of protein powder and Carboplex to the communal collection in the kitchen, All the while, I endured their silent stares, which did not relent until we sat down for lunch.

"So you've just joined *Shangwi-La,* huh?" Bamm Bamm finally asked, his chair groaning from his bulk. There was something about the way he said Shangri-La, that made me wonder. It wasn't the lisp that was the giveaway. It was his tone of voice—it sounded like he hated it. And sure enough, he did. All three of them did.

As I discovered from my new friends, Shangri-La had replaced Bill Pearl's gym which had stood for years just a few blocks away. Pearl's was as legendary as its owner. It offered heavy weights in abundance and large humans wanting to get larger. According to Nimrod and Bamm Bamm, its other advantages included a spyhole to the women's locker room and the tanning bed.

But Shangri-La was another kettle of fish altogether, calling itself not a gym but a fitness training center, offering not only weights, but an aerobics floor, motivational business seminars, dietary counseling and child care. The difference lay in the personality of the owners. Or, as Nimrod put it succinctly, "Bill Pearl is Bill Pearl, man, Raoul is Raoul."

From what I could gather from the bitter talk at the table, Bill Pearl was pro-building, Raoul pro-business. Pearl, the greatest body-builder in the world in his time, built because he had to. It was an essential part of his soul. He was simply diseased; his daily workouts, which began at four A.M., were a symptom. His gym catered to men and women similarly stricken, every workout offering the opportunity for a fistfight and the "Heightened Arousal Mode."

But as bodybuilding became conventional in the eighties, embraced and endorsed by Yuppies across the land, Raoul had latched onto it as a business opportunity and a vehicle for his ego. He sold motivational posters of himself, car shades, key rings, booklets bearing his image, and his own line of weight-lifting wear. He even stopped working out, believing it no longer "cost-effective." Instead, he could be found glued to the personal computer in his back office, directing the flow of merchandise. To my new friends, Raoul was shameless, since his body—at its best not in the world's top one hundred—wasn't worth the merchandising. Bill Pearl, with so much more to offer, wasn't interested in selling it. One was a profiteer, the other a purist. That explained Raoul's braces. It also explained builders vs. the world, what I had witnessed at the gym. To hard-core bodybuilders like Vinnie, Nimrod, and Bamm Bamm, the gym was no longer a refuge. Since I was a muscle parvenu, my new friends had to know where I stood. This would be tough, but not impossible.

"So, where do *you* come from?" Nimrod asked gruffly.

"New York's from New York," Vinnie responded.

Nimrod looked at Vinnie. "He can speak for himself, can't he?"

"Yes, he can," I said, basso profundo.

From the other side of the table, Bamm Bamm fired his salvo, "My dad's in the tool and die business, what about yours?"

In good bodybuilding tradition, I paused and thought before giving an appropriate response. I couldn't very well pipe up and say, "Oh, he's a literary and cultural critic, perhaps you're familiar with his latest—it's just out in paper, you know, *The Rhetorical World of Augustan Humanism?*" No, that wouldn't do. I had to find something stronger, something nobler.

"He's dead," I said.

"Was he a lifter?" Nimrod asked suspiciously, pausing with his fork at his mouth.

I was in over my head, but I couldn't stop now. "He certainly was," I lied. "His name was Tug. He was so massive, they buried him in a piano case and lowered the casket into the grave by crane." I assuaged my guilt by reminding myself that a bodybuilder's fundamental task is reinvention.

Vinnie came to my defense and settled the matter. "Hey, Big Man's all right," he said, annoyed, "you should have seen him throw up this morning after squats."

This was just what Bamm Bamm and Nimrod wanted to hear. All three of them retired to their rooms. A few minutes later, Bamm Bamm and Nimrod returned bearing disposable syringes and glass vials.

"Dessert," Bamm Bamm explained, dropping his trousers and underwear as Nimrod filled an upturned 3-cc syringe with yellow liquid he drew from a vial. It looked remarkably like urine.

Nimrod withdrew the needle from the vial, slapped Bamm Bamm's naked ass once, then plunged the syringe an inch and a half deep into Bamm Bamm's flesh.

"Grow, grow, grow," Nimrod murmured, working the plunger.

"Jesus, *Nimwod*, it feels like a fuckin' garden hose. Are you sure that's a new one?" Bamm Bamm asked querulously.

I thought I was going to faint. Just then, Vinnie came into the living room, and said in concern: "What, Sam, this isn't new, is it?"

Nimrod looked over in my direction, his face visibly brightening. When he pulled the steel dart out of Bamm Bamm's ass, the tiny hole spurted forth a stream of blood which landed with a splat on the plastic-covered sofa. "Nimrod, Bamm Bamm, one of you get the Windex, OK?" In deference to guests, Vinnie explained to me.

That very day, Vinnie began my education as a bodybuilder and instructed me on the merits of performance-enhancing drugs. Drugs were an essential part of "the physique agenda," as he called it, as integral to success for a truly committed builder as hard training and a good diet. And at 1404 Delacey, one could expect these "shooting parties" every afternoon. Didn't I know? Vinnie asked. As far as drugs were concerned, all my bodybuilding heroes were on everything but roller skates.

I knew nothing, but I'd *heard* everything. Both in his autobiography and on talk shows, Arnold admitted his steroid use with a mischievous chuckle. But Arnold could afford to laugh, he had retired. For the current crop of world-class bodybuilders, steroids were a nonsubject. But if the bodybuilding community clammed up on steroids, there was no shortage of juice yarns among lesser lifters. Rumors of "'roid rage" drifted through every gym. It was said to be a violent, psychotic condition linked to testosterone intake. I knew that in Maryland a thief had even won a jury's sympathy by claiming "the steroid defense." If it didn't excuse his series of nocturnal neighborhood robberies and assaults, at least it explained it.

From what the newspapers said, these drugs had been around since the early fifties for medical patients suffering adrenal insufficiency, certain types of anemia, and massive tissue loss. But in 1958, Dr. John Ziegler, a physician for the U.S. weight-lifting team, developed with the Ciba pharmaceutical company America's first anabolic steroid specifically designed for strength athletes. They christened their wonder drug Dianabol (in the gym, it's abbreviated as D-ball).

In the sixties and early seventies steroids were the secret of strength athletes. It was the lifters and shotputters and discus throwers of the world who used the drugs. But word got around, and by the mid-seventies steroids had found their way to the training table of professional and college football players. By the late eighties steroid use had exploded. Studies showed that 6 percent of high school students and 15 to 20 percent of college athletes *admitted* taking steroids. Football, tennis, cross-country skiing, track and field, swimming, even fencing—no sport was immune. But it was in bodybuilding, the only sport that relies exclusively on muscle mass for judgment, the drugs worked best, and bodybuilders have been using them since the days of Dr. Ziegler.

Vinnie took time out from what he called his "import/export business" to educate me personally in this matter. Being on the juice, or taking steroids, or, as some lifters call it, "taking shit," simply meant that the builder was using either synthetic male hormone of an oral variety or an injectable one. Whether you swallow it or inject it, the drug eventually finds its way into the bloodstream where it spots muscle cells and attaches itself to receptor sites within each cell. The result? An increased level of protein synthesis within each cell, which, over time, means greater muscles and faster recuperation for the lifter.

No, I couldn't count on 30 or 40 pounds of muscle gain over a few months, as articles in *Sports Illustrated* suggested (the same articles that spoke so vividly of "'roid rage"). But if I trained like a wild man and ate voraciously, I could count on at least 10 and maybe 15 pounds of muscle gain (much of it in the form of water retention) over the same period of time.

Vinnie led me into his own room to continue my education. The placed looked like a Federal Express terminal, filled with plain brown envelopes and cardboard containers of all sizes. Vinnie's business, he readily admitted, was steroids. At the foot of his bed was his "treasure chest," as he called it, a footlocker holding scores of magical growth enhancers in bottle and vial form. I couldn't believe the sheer variety of pharmaceutical options available to those involved in the pursuit of muscular accretion. A whole new world opened up to me filled with mystical names and properties.

Names like Finajet, Dihydrotest, testosterone cypionate, An-adrol, Deca, Esclene, Lasix, Dianabol, Halotestin, Blastron. They sounded like city-states in a science fiction novel. Maxibol, Pri-moteston Depot 100, Proviron, Sostenon 250, Cytomel. There were drugs that increased your strength, drugs that decreased your body fat, drugs that ballooned the muscle for just a few hours, drugs that altered your mood.

Vinnie saved the best for last. He lovingly cradled in his hands a large bottle that contained a liquid substance known as human growth hormone. It had been extracted from the pituitary glands of cadavers. It was sweet stuff, said Vinnie, used by all bodybuilding greats in the 8-week countdown before a contest. Excessive use, of course, promoted an unsightly enlargement of the jaw and forehead, the mysterious appearance of a gap between the two front teeth, the irreversible growth of the extremities (including the genitals), and, occasionally, sudden death. But it was just these possibilities, Vinnie added with a wild look, that made human growth hormone, or HGH, the ultimate test of a builder's commitment.

It wasn't just HGH that could be followed by bad news, though—at least according to the white slip of paper that fell to the floor from one of Vinnie's vials. In my hands, the sheet folded out like an accordion, and I read the fine print of the manufacturer's warning detailing the negative effects from undergoing any form of what Vinnie grandly called "steroid therapy."

A condition called gynecomastia was one (what Tony, back at the Juice Bar, had called "gyno" that morning). It was more com-monly known in the gym as "bitch tits," in which the victim suffers a bulbous swelling under one or both nipples—the body's estrogen reaction to counteract the flood of testosterone. Take a good look in the magazines at the best bodybuilders, the Mr. Olympia con-tenders, Vinnie suggested, and you'll find quite a selection of big builders sporting the telltale tumor.

But all was not lost, he assured me. A drug called Nolvadex could be taken to counteract the original drug that created the condition. The jury was still out on the possible side effects of Nolvadex.

And there were other little problems from the drugs, the sheet said, problems like premature baldness, lowered sperm count, increased body hair, rectal bleeding, dizzy spells, thyroid and liver and kidney malfunction, gallstones, cancer, gastrointestinal upset, hepatitis, raised levels of aggression ("'roid rage" again), and, of course, acne. I noticed that Vinnie himself suffered from the latter malady, and asked him if his skin condition was related to his steroid-supplementation program.

"You know, Sam, I think muscles are worth a few zits, don't you?" he asked.

I watched as Vinnie delved into his treasure chest and emerged with a small box of one hundred white pills, a syringe, and two vials for me. Vinnie prescribed four Anavar pills after breakfast and four more after dinner. They should never be taken on an empty stomach, he warned, or I might get ulcers. Eight of these per day for the next eight weeks, along with two shots per week of injectables ought to break my plateau quite nicely.

Each injection consisted of 2 ccs of Deca and 1 cc of testosterone cypionate. The testosterone and Deca (the bread-and-butter drug of bodybuilders) would work well for my strength and weight gain. The Anavar, combined with what Vinnie called "an intelligent diet," would help me get cut (or defined).

As I lowered my trousers and underwear, and bared my ass cheek, I tried to fight off my fear of needles by concentrating on the financial aspects of the operation. Vinnie charged me "wholesale prices" for the drugs: I bought four Anavar bottles (one hundred pills each) at $25.00 a bottle; sixteen 2-cc vials of Deca at $5.00 each, and two 10-cc vials of testosterone cypionate at $20.00 apiece. My first eight-week cycle cost $220.00 (prices vary according to how many hands touch the drugs before you do). But when Vinnie neared with the inch and a half syringe, my jaw dropped. Was I taking too much too soon?

Not to worry, said Vinnie. True, I was "stacking" on my first "cycle," that is, taking more than one drug at a time on my eight- to ten-week program. But he had been "shotgunning" for years, inundating his body with all kinds of quantities in all kinds of combinations in the hope that his body hadn't built an immunity to them all. Nimrod and Bamm Bamm did the same, and they were still standing, weren't they? They were in fact, just then, watching and giggling a few feet away.

"You're a big man, Sam," Vinnie said, silencing me with a look, "and big men take big cycles. That's how they get real big." I waited for the inevitable, and, sure enough, it came. "Besides, that which doesn't kill you makes you stronger."

I only hoped to God that which made me stronger didn't kill me. I yelped as Vinnie plunged the needle attached to a plastic, disposable syringe into me. It felt as thick as a finger. My gluteus muscles began to fibrillate helplessly in shock.

I told myself that taking steroids was a Faustian bargain. I was selling my soul to the devil in exchange for transcending what was permitted to ordinary mortals. I was my own alchemist, I said, transmuting the base metal of myself, the dross, into gold. To the diseased, there is no pyrite.

It was intensely personal, but I could deal with it only abstractly. To bodybuild without steroids was to read Russian literature in translation, I said, rubbing my hand over my swollen, twitching bottom. I even invoked the transitive property of equality: bodybuilding and muscular growth are synonymous; steroids and muscular growth are synonymous; therefore bodybuilding and steroids are synonymous.

When faced with the syringe, even my own worst fears didn't matter. I couldn't stop. Seventeen-inch arms were not enough; I wanted 20. And when I got to 20, I was sure that I'd want 22. My retreat to the weight room was a retreat into the simple world of numbers. Numerical gradations were the only thing left in my life that made sense. Twenty was better than 17, but worse than 22. Bench pressing 315 was better than bench pressing 275, but worse than 365. I was reduced to a world where such thinking ruled, and it was only by embracing it that I could sleep at night.

Besides, I was desperate. If who you are is what you do, and as a bodybuilder, what you do is what you look like, then in California I was distinctly in trouble, because I didn't look like a bodybuilder. Not after two years of training. Not compared to Vinnie or Nimrod, much less Raoul, or even Lamar.

And as long as I didn't look like a builder, I wasn't comfortable with myself. Delivering my muscle lines was not enough. Mr. World, Tom Platz, was quoted in *USA Today* as saying he first took steroids because in competitions, "you get tired of finishing second." I was concerned far less with competition than with self-identity. I needed to complete my transformation. As long as the part I played was simply interior, I felt like a fraud. No, I needed the juice in the worst way, to make myself whole. I needed to complete the new persona, to make myself into a bodybuilder.

When Vinnie reached into his footlocker to get some blue Dianabol pills and a syringe for himself, he confided to me of lean times back in New York, when he had fled from life with the help of cocaine and the bottle.

"Yeah, Sam, after a few years with AA and other support groups, I got off the drugs and alcohol, and I ain't never looked back," he said. I watched as he plunged 3 ccs of Deca Durabolin into his own ass cheek. I was startled by the state of Vinnie's bottom. It looked like an aerial shot of Ypres, circa 1917, with great craters here, trenches there, everywhere physical bombardment. Vinnie noticed my look of alarm and explained his condition.

"It's scar tissue, Sam, from the injections," he said, chuckling at my reaction. "You know, sometimes I get little knots in my ass. And when I push the needle in, it hits a knot and bounces right on out. Hell, you play the game, you pay the price, but no problem, you can't see the scars when I'm wearin' my posin' trunks, so the judges can't take off no points. Every few months, you know, in a periodical fashion, I go to a surgeon, and he removes a knot or two."

As he spoke, I watched the blood seep out from my recent puncture wound to spread through the fabric of my underwear. Despite my resolve, I felt sick to my stomach.

8.

THE DIGS

WHAT PEOPLE SAW WHEN HE APPEARED BEFORE THEM, THEN, WAS NOT REALLY HIM, BUT A PERSON HE HAD INVENTED, AN ARTIFICIAL CREATURE HE COULD MANIPULATE IN ORDER TO MANIPULATE OTHERS. HE HIMSELF REMAINED INVISIBLE, A PUPPETEER WORKING THE STRINGS OF HIS ALTER-EGO FROM A DARK, SOLITARY PLACE BEHIND THE CURTAIN.

——PAUL AUSTER

I had come to California knowing I would take steroids. But I hadn't expected to be on them by my second day. From the very start, I relied on "the juice" to give me two things I sorely lacked after only two and a half years of lifting; thickness and "muscle maturity." The thickness lessons I'd taken at the Y had been a start, but if it weren't for steroids, I'd need at least three more years to really get thick. As for "muscle maturity," that's the polish, the sheen, the finish in the form of deep-muscle separation and definition that comes with a half-decade of training. A half-decade, that is, unless one resorts to the juice. And I, for one, couldn't wait three or four or five more years to become myself. I was so uncomfortable not being "me" that I had to have it, now.

I took that first injection in October of 1986 and within two months, I had gained 15 pounds on my first cycle. Much of it was water retention; my body shape remained the same, but I didn't notice that. What I noticed was that the scale read 245 pounds. The plateau had finally been shattered. As long as I stuffed myself with my bodybuilding foods and swallowed my eight Anavar pills a day, and twice a week endured my testosterone and Deca injections, I could count on not losing a pound. At least, I hoped that was what I was taking. Because of the extraordinary demand, the market was flooded with bogus steroids. Retailers not uncommonly substituted pills of aspirin for Anavar, and replaced vials of legitimate steroids with vegetable and sesame seed oil. Builders call them blanks.

But judging by my gains, both in strength and bodyweight, my source was pure. My bench press increased from a 1-rep best of 315 to 405 pounds in six months. I went from benching 275 for eight to 365 for eight. My squat increased from 405 to 545. Bent over rows from 225 to 315, dumbbell curls from 60 to 75.

The heavier weight I lifted forced my body to respond. Pumping out 10 reps with 225 pounds on the incline bench is a strain, but 10 reps with 315 pounds is much more of a strain. Now that I was capable of the latter, my body had no choice but to grow.

In six short weeks I was no longer the smallest resident of 1404 Delacey. Almost before my eyes, my arms gained half an inch, my thighs three-quarters of an inch, my neck a full inch. It wasn't long before I surpassed Nimrod on all the major strength exercises in the gym. Soon after that, I overtook Vinnie himself.

But while I looked better and better, I began to feel worse and worse. Headaches were a daily affair. And I *worried*. Among the many 'roid rumors, there were some unmistakable facts. In 1984, for instance, weight-lifting great Paul Anderson underwent a kidney transplant. In 1987, Mr. America, Dave Johns, a notorious juicer, died from what physicians termed "a mysterious fever." Professional bodybuilder Dave Draper suffered a massive coronary, Tom Platz endured the ignominy of gallstones.

If the health reports from the field were staggering, they could always be explained away—at least by my fellow gym rats. Studies have found that steroids lead to an increased risk of heart disease, I whispered nervously. Well, yes, but is it the steroids, or all that stuffing of food and sudden weight gain, they rebutted. There seems to be a link between steroids and that psychotic emotional condition known as " 'roid rage," I mentioned, as casually as possible. Well yes, my muscular friends replied, but is it the steroids, or the frame of mind a lifter has to have to lift inhuman quantities of weight?

The more I researched the steroid results, the more I understood their answers. To date, it is all a gray, murky zone, untested and unproven. As Dr. James C. Puffer, head physician for the U.S. team in the 1988 Olympics Games, has admitted: "We don't know as much as we pretend to know." There are far more questions about the drug than answers, mainly because in the few experiments done in the past, doctors have had difficulty getting athletes to take just the prescribed doses. As we might imagine by now, the builders have had a tendency to do *more*. . . .

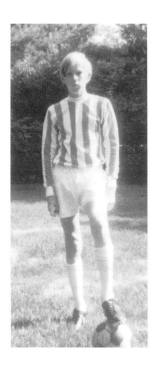

PRE-IRON

◁ Author, age fourteen, in soccer uniform

▽ Age twenty-two

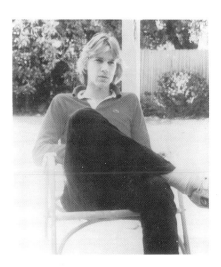

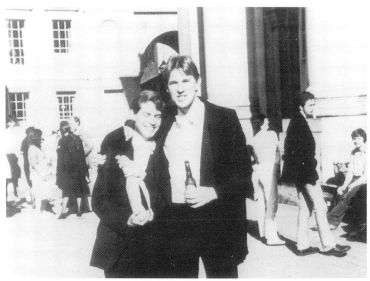

Age twenty-four, celebrating the conclusion of Oxford examinations

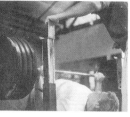 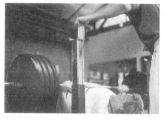 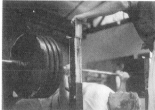

The descent   The pause   The explosion

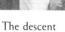
Author squatting 405 pounds

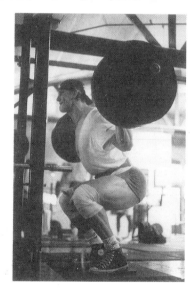

Squatting 500 pounds

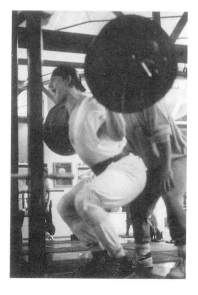

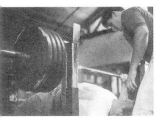 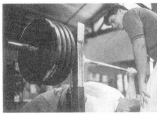 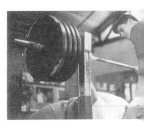

The explosion (continued)   The initial phase of lockout   The lockout

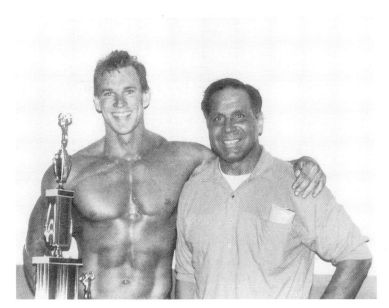

Author with bodybuilding great Bill Pearl at the San Gabriel Valley

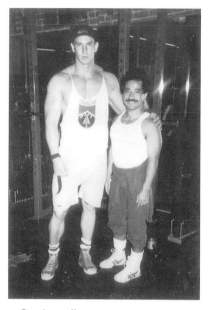

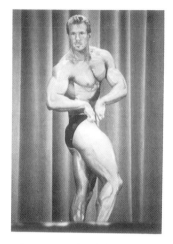

On stage at the Golden Valley

△ Standing tall
with Hero Isagawa,
current bench-press
world record holder
for the 123-pound
weight class

Author ▷
rubbing his chin
(post "Heightened
Arousal Mode") at
the Ninth Annual
Rose City Bench-Press
Extravaganza

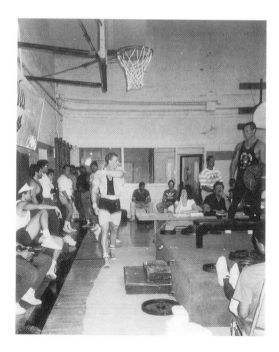

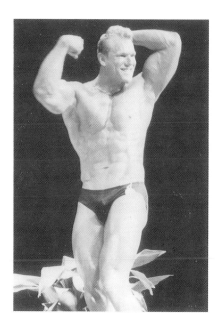

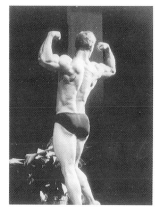

△ The compulsory back
double-biceps pose at the
San Gabriel Valley
◁ Doing "Hair" at the
San Gabriel Valley

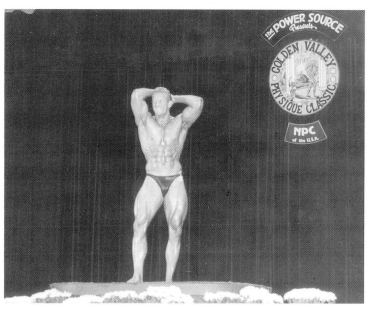

Abdominal pose at the Golden Valley

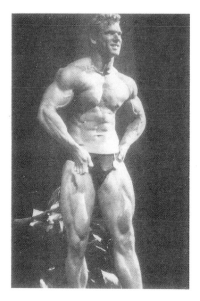

◁ Holding water at the
San Gabriel Valley

▽ After "the Diet"—
six days later, 12 pounds lighter
at the Golden Valley

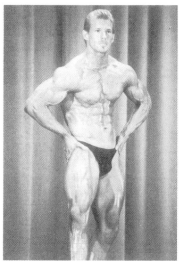

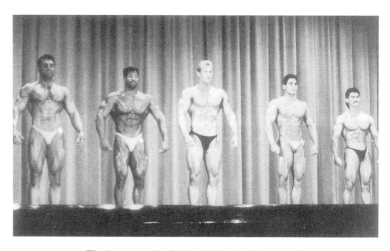

The lineup at the Golden Valley (author center)

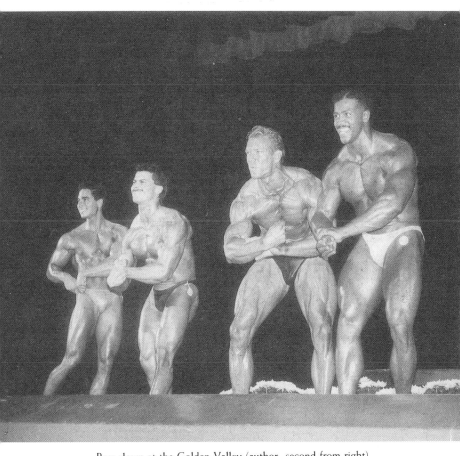

Pose-down at the Golden Valley (author, second from right)

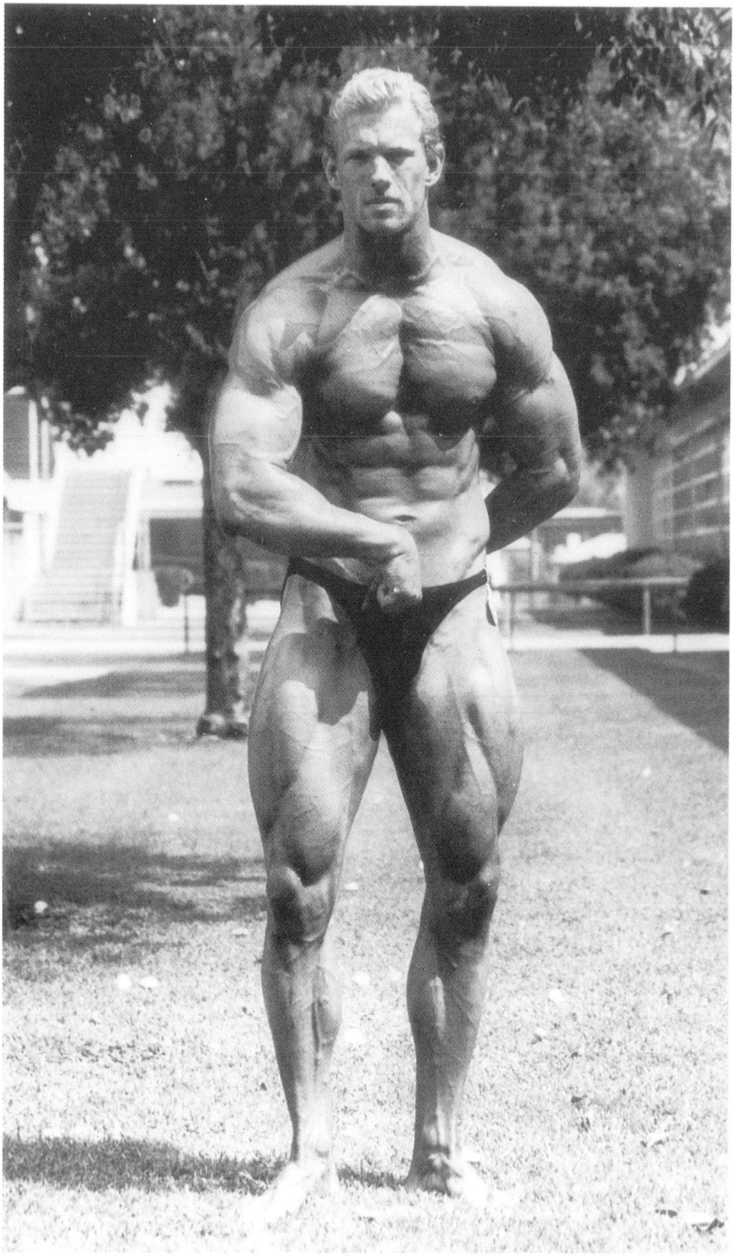

John R. Coletti © 1991

A bodybuilder at last. Author, 1988.

And to bodybuilders—save for the renegade physicians who still prescribed steroids—the medical community as a whole was not to be trusted. After all, for over a decade the American College of Sports Medicine had officially maintained that steroids didn't work, that they failed to increase muscle mass. The fact was that they did. Vinnie and Bamm Bamm and Nimrod could all attest to that. The question was: What else did they do? From October of 1986 to September of 1988, I found out for myself.

The rectal bleeding, I passed off as just a consequence of my deep squatting technique. Vinnie always made fun of his own hemorrhoids, calling attention to what he called "flippers" that seemed to emerge, crawling and quivering with life, from the site of the discomfort. But rectal bleeding could always be hidden with Vinnie's Huggies.

It was the acne I couldn't hide. As the months flew by and I trained and ate and injected, the acne invasion spread from my face to my neck, my chest, my upper back, even my scalp, until, finally, it found its way to my shins and toes. Wherever I had skin, I had pimples.

But the biggest pain was in my ass. It ached constantly from my twice weekly injections. For weeks on end, a bad shot left a knot, a fist-sized tightening and swelling. The only proper way to receive the syringe was to relax the ass cheek and jab the needle in quickly, all the way to the base. But I had a tendency to tighten my gluteus muscles in fear. The result? A bruise the size of a pomegranate. Vinnie laughed at my problems, advising me not to wear tights. I learned to sit down very gingerly.

I was grateful that, even though I had increased my dosage significantly, I hadn't yet begun to grow bald like Nimrod or Bamm Bamm. And though I checked every so often during the course of the day, I could not detect the beginning of a bitch-tit lurking beneath either nipple. Soreness, yes. An actual bulb, no.

The reaction wasn't just physical. I found myself psychologically affected as well. Judging by my behavior, I had to admit that self-defense was no longer my muscle motive. Now, out on the sidewalk or in line at the movie theater, sitting in the park or standing at the bank, I needed to rule. Self-preservation had metamorphosed into something quite beyond self-publication. The T-shirts and tank tops and body language I'd used back in New York no longer sufficed.

I was fueled by my own anger, which I seemed to draw from an inexhaustible source. I watched almost as a spectator as my body operated beyond my control. I wasn't just aching for a fist fight, I was begging for it. I longed for the release. So I strutted through the city streets, a juggernaut in a do-rag, glaring and menacing anyone who dared meet my eye. On the road, I was no better than Vinnie. Any motorist ahead of me drove too slowly, and I tailgated them mercilessly to teach them a lesson. Anyone behind me drove too fast, and I cured them of tailgating by grinding Vinnie's bastard barge to a complete halt, shaking in nervous excitement behind the wheel in anticipation of blows. The shouting matches invariably ended as soon as I discarded my shirt for battle. My opponents always fled.

In calmer moments, my behavior baffled and frightened me, but Vinnie understood it at once. "Shit, Big Man, that's just takin' charge," he explained. "Ain't nothin' wrong with that. Do you think the cowboys *asked* the Injuns for their land? You bet your ass they didn't. They just shot 'em and took it, right?"

To him, my "attitude" was perfect. To take charge, as he put it, whenever and wherever possible was the natural state of things. I was like a shark, he said. It made my motives sound almost pure.

Little solace that would have been to the man I encountered in the supermarket on Fair Oaks Avenue. Toupee and all, he quibbled with the cashier over twenty cents on an item purchased. The argument lasted over three minutes while the rest of us in line waited silently behind him. Finally, I couldn't wait another second.

"GET THE FUCK OUT OF HERE!" I screamed at the man. "YOU'RE HOLDING US BACK!" I yelled, as if the issue concerned muscular growth. The man didn't utter a sound. His face turned white, and holding his rug to his scalp, he fled.

In the gym, I was even worse. I refused to let others work in with me while I did my exercises. Time was, a cheer and a nod from me would welcome them, but not now. Not when I spent the 45 seconds between my sets stalking and pacing nervously by the

131 · THE DIGS

equipment. I resented even the passage of time for delaying my next set.

From my first moment on the juice, nothing else mattered. Nothing but my workouts, my growth, my meals, my injections, and my friends, who were concerned with their workouts, their growth, their meals, their injections. Everything else was not just secondary—it was positively inconsequential.

"ISOLATE!" Vinnie screamed at me in the gym as the months passed. "ISOLATE!"

He was referring to the technique known as "Muscle Isolation," maximizing growth by blocking out distractions and concentrating only on the muscle at hand. So I thought only of my biceps or my triceps or my deltoids or my calves during workouts. But we could have been anywhere at any time, because "Muscle Isolation" didn't stop in the gym.

Back at 1404 Delacey, we builders were nothing if not isolated, sequestered in willful disobedience against the rest of the world, and steroids were our agents of divorce. It was us against them, bodybuilders against mankind. Our home was like a sumo wrestler's stable. In place of the *mawashi* (the ceremonial diaper), the *geta* (wooden sandals), and the formal kimona worn by the sumotori outside the stable, we wrapped ourselves in our layers of Gold's Gym clothes. They defined who we were and what we did as clearly as our refusal to eat restaurant food (where meat might suffer the taint of salt or fish the sacrilege of butter). The sumotori stuffed themselves with their sacred *chankonabe* (boiled fish or meat, vegetables and seaweed), while we downed our chicken breasts, fish, yams, dry noodles, and defatted beef in the privacy of our refuge.

But we shared more than vestments and diet and sequestration. In both sports, posture was half the performance. Measuring his opponent in the ring, the sumo wrestler goes through his ritual: the rice fling, the foot stomp, the stare, the restless shifting into position, the eventual contact. The mirror in the gym, the lifting belt, the ammonia, the slap, the scream, the lift—bodybuilding was not much different. For Vinnie, for Nimrod, for Bamm Bamm, for me, it was an existence so stylized it left room for little else. That was the point.

"EAT BIG, SLEEP BIG, TRAIN BIG" was the iron edict obeyed by all of us. In our muscle stable, we averaged 5,000 calories a day. The stove was constantly burning, the oven baking, the refrigerator cooling, the cupboards storing. The preparation of food, the storing of food, the consumption of food, the elimination of food. "You can't grow unless you eat" is a bodybuilding maxim that we at 1404 Delacey proved true. Nimrod injected himself on a daily basis with vitamin B_{12} in order to maintain his extraordinary appetite. Vinnie could be heard throwing up every afternoon from an excess of food even his body couldn't take. Considering the frequency and volume with which Bamm Bamm ate, it was a wonder that he weighed only 290 pounds.

To us, food represented fuel for the future. Every chicken breast and beef flank we ate was consumed in the hope that it would help make us into the giants we dreamed of being. A few chicken helpings more, and we were that much closer to turning our dreams into reality.

The toll of all this food and two daily workouts with heavy, heavy weight was a chronic need for rest. Such, in fact, was the demand of the discipline that we were incapable of doing *anything* else. At Oxford, I'd gotten by on six hours of sleep at night. Here in Southern California, I found I needed twelve just to make it through the day, and my friends were no different.

We saved most of our dreaming for our waking hours, the afternoon hours the three of us spent in the living room practicing our posing. Surfers dream of the perfect wave, builders of the perfect 90 seconds of posing. In bodybuilding competitions, the 90 seconds are called "the free posing round."

For just one minute and a half, the builder glides on the dais to the musical composition of his or her choice. Vinnie was still misty-eyed over his last performance at the Southwestern Connecticut State Bodybuilding Championship. As he reminisced (and not for the first time), "Let me just say one thing, guys, it was as good as an erection. There I was, on stage in my posing oil and black trunks, and the crowd really loved me. I mean I *moved* 'em with my posing exhibition. It was just my fuckin' time."

All of my roommates had competed, and with their help, I

learned not only the standard poses, like the front double-biceps and the back-lat spread, but the accepted variations, like the Farnese *Hercules* and Michelangelo's *David*. Bodybuilders have used the postures of classical and renaissance sculpture for effect since Sandow at the beginning of the twentieth century. The Farnese *Hercules* included one foot forward and one foot back, one arm in front of the body at hip level and one arm behind, a tightening of the torso and a pensive look downward. *David* involved a hip shift to the right with a corresponding move of bodyweight onto the right leg. From there, the right hand held at the right thigh, the left arm held up near the shoulder (as if holding the dreaded sling), and a look of nobility to the left. Every afternoon, we resembled a parodic tableau vivant, mechanically moving in and out of our poses.

But while my three friends delighted in their posing, I couldn't quite stomach it. It was no problem for me to make myself a living statue. It was a problem to believe in it. No matter how I figured it, the fundamental purpose of a posing routine seemed to be to encapsulate and reduce life to 90 ticking seconds. Somehow, it rankled me; it seemed *wrong*. As wrong, in its own way, as bullying people out on the street. As wrong as subscribing to that other act of life-reduction so favored by Xandra and Vinnie and Lamar: the motto. No matter how hard I tried, I couldn't eradicate my skepticism.

The magazines didn't help. My roommates spent their few non-lifting, non-eating, non-sleeping hours reading them, pausing every so often to announce what they would do when they were discovered by "Joe."

To them and the rest of the bodybuilding community, "Joe" meant Joe Weider, the muscle publisher, impresario and self-proclaimed "Master Blaster," the one-time grocery delivery boy and short-order cook who had parlayed his teenage lifting fanaticism into a publishing empire. With over 2,000 employees, his business grosses more than $250 million a year.

His magazines include *Muscle & Fitness*, *Shape*, *Flex*, *Men's Fitness*, and, yes, *Moxie*. Joe Weider sponsored and created the greatest bodybuilding contest, the Mr. Olympia. He cofounded with his brother Ben the International Federation of Bodybuilders (the dominant professional league) with 136 member countries. He brought Arnold to America and kept a limited number of builders on salary.

But I knew even more about Joe. Unlike my friends, I had different sources, the daily newspapers and weekly newsmagazines, and I knew that this same Joe had recently shelled out $400,000 to the Federal Trade Commission for an out-of-court settlement involving his "Anabolic Mega-Pak" and his "Dynamic Life Essence" pills. According to the United States government, they were not the surefire muscle growers advertised in his magazines.

And there was more. While his magazine *Muscle & Fitness* belabors the point that bodybuilding really has nothing to do with vanity, Joe Weider's name can be found well over two hundred times in every issue. It's everywhere, from the front cover to the labels of the products advertised in its pages, from the trophies the builders hold in the photos to the glowing testimonials entitled "My Friend Joe Weider."

Issue after issue of *Muscle & Fitness* presented my roommates with the same photograph of an awe-inspiring bust of Joe, their Joe. But I had read that Joe admitted that the bust was a sham. The muscular torso, the swollen arms, everything beneath the collarbone, in fact, belonged to IFBB competitor Robby Robinson. Only the face belonged to Joe, and by 1990 it was in sorry sagging shape.

My roommates ignored the Joe who, under attack, defended himself by saying Jesus and Moses had had their detractors too. It never seemed to occur to them that most of the articles in Joe's magazines were simply advertising spiels for the protein products and arm blasters found in the pages that followed.

I didn't draw it to their attention, but it was hard not to notice these facts myself. To my roommates, Ben Weider, brother of Joe, was a brilliant bodybuilding administrator. But I had read that Ben had a passion for Napoleonic memorabilia, including, in his private collection, a priceless lock of Bonaparte's hair. If that isn't a warning sign, what is?

The newspapers I read were also a valuable asset in shedding light on other heroes in the muscle magazines. In *Muscle & Fitness*, Sergio Oliva was one of the greatest Mr. Olympias the world has ever known. In the newspapers, he was dissuaded from beating his battered wife to a pulp only by a few well-aimed shots triggered by her from his own revolver. In the hagiography of the muscle magazines, Dennis Tinerino was Mr. Universe. In the black-and-white print of the newspapers, he was arrested and jailed for pandering.

I didn't tell my roommates that my Joe and Ben and Sergio and Dennis were one and the same as theirs. I saw no reason to infect them with my knowledge. The fact that I knew it was awful enough, since once I perceived it, I couldn't very well pretend that none of it mattered, any more than I could pretend that those "'roid rages" of mine on the road and in the grocery store were cowboy and Indian fun.

I felt I had to know more about my muscle crusade. It no longer seemed so noble or defensible a proposition as I'd once thought. In the gym, I was fine because it was the one place on earth I was safe from the perils of thought. But Lamar and Vinnie, Nimrod and Bamm Bamm, diapers and baby food, demands and rages? Was I, too, a case of arrested development, caught in a perpetual nightmare of adolescence? Or, despite everything, was I judging too hastily? What had led them to iron and why did they stick it out, burrowing ever deeper into the gym world? If a man is known by the company he keeps, what kind of company was I keeping? I felt that if I could learn a little more about them, I might learn a little more about myself.

Thus I found myself wandering back to the rooms of my roommates. "Nimrod," I asked, "what led you to iron?"

"When I graduated from junior high," Nimrod recalled fondly, "Dad gave me my first weights, a bench-press set and a squat rack."

I remembered my own eighth grade graduation. My father had proudly presented me with a full reference library consisting of fifty bulky leather-bound volumes.

"Since then," Nimrod said, "I ain't never looked back. From 125 to 280."

"280?" I asked. Nimmy was large, but because of his year-round ripped condition, not that large. Two hundred forty would have been stretching it.

"Two hundred eighty," he said, leading me into his room.

As I crossed the threshold, the first thing that struck me was

The Work. The only decoration in the room, it hung above the waterbed. All the other walls were bare. I tiptoed around the magazines carelessly strewn on the floor to examine a king-sized sheet nailed to the wall. On its white surface, Nimrod had painstakingly painted the number 280. This was the only mark on the sheet. An open bucket of wet black paint with a brush in it lay beneath The Work. The individual numbers were raised a full inch off the cotton surface, like welts, from so many repeated coatings.

"Two eighty, that's my goal for January first, 280."

I didn't know what to say. I came out with "Don't serve time, make time serve you." I'd heard it in the gym. It seemed appropriate.

But Nimrod didn't hear a thing. He only had eyes for his sheet, and before long he mechanically moved to the wall, stooped to pick up the brush, then set about repeating his applications. As he labored, he told me of his affiliation with the University of Florida. Nimrod hadn't actually been a student there, but that hadn't prevented him from living on campus. In the women's dorms exclusively. In fact, Nimrod had spent four full years servicing the sororities of the University of Florida. As he said, "It beats dieting for a contest, eh?"

"You must have been a busy man," I said wistfully. I hadn't been that busy in well over a year. My New York girlfriend had jilted me for her fiancé. "What's your secret?" I asked.

He closed the door. "Hydrogen peroxide, extensions, and contacts," he whispered.

I looked at him, baffled.

"Once a week I take a teaspoon of hydrogen peroxide with my water. It clears up the skin," he confessed.

As for his hair, those long gleaming blond locks were made of dyed nylon. "Extensions," he called them. They were strands of hair actually anchored and woven into his own dark roots. At last I understood why Nimrod was the only builder I knew without that scraggly scattering of hair known as the "picket fence" look, so common among heavy steroid users.

Nimrod completed "the package," as he called himself, with his contact lenses, which were colored to make his brown eyes blue.

"Aside from that, it's the muscles. Jesus, do you know how many chicks I've pulled thanks to this?" he said, flexing, then staring in admiration at his engorged bicep.

"Big Man Muscles," I said, parroting Vinnie.

"Hey, if you seen me pumped up in the gym, you don't think I'm no *man!*" He spat out the word in disgust. "You'd think I was, like, a race horse, yeah, one of those gleaming thoroughbreds with my blond mane whistling in the wind. I don't look like no *guy*. I don't want to look like no *guy*.

"Look here," he said, "how many inches you got?" I wasn't sure how to interpret this and hemmed and hawed until Nimrod grabbed my upper arm.

"Oh, that . . . uh, 18," I estimated.

"Hanging?" He meant with my arm simply lying limp, not flexed.

"About 17," I admitted.

"See, I got 20 inches hanging and the way I train, these babies are here to stay. I want to look like something you've never seen before."

I understood. The shock value is all. It's saying, or rather screaming, "More than anything else in the world, whatever it takes, I don't want to be like you. I don't want to look like you, I don't want to talk like you, I don't want to *be* you."

I forbore to suggest my own theory to Nimrod: that bodybuilding, decorating the body to such an extreme, was a principally feminine exercise (not to mention the extensions and contacts). He wouldn't have heard me even if I had.

He'd wandered back with his brush to the sheet and was busy applying more coats. It didn't matter to him what he looked like at 280 pounds. He just wanted to get there, stay there, then diet down from there for a contest. It was a very sad day for us all at 1404 Delacey when, months later, Nimrod tearfully painted over the upper portion of his 8 to alter it to a 6. He felt it was more realistic. We felt that someone had died in the family.

I hated to admit it even to myself, but there was something about what Nimrod had said about hating to be human that rang a bell inside me. It wasn't that I wanted to be a dog or a cat or even a dolphin or, as in Nimrod's case, a horse. Their lives seemed far worse than mine. It was just that I didn't see much about being human that I liked either. Pre-iron, I'd spent my days convicting myself of avarice and envy and sloth. To become something else seemed the only alternative. As long as I covered myself with the equivalent of scaffolding and labeled myself a "work in progress," I could escape the doubt and uncertainty that plagued my past and spend every second of my present concentrating on a pristine future. I hated the flawed, weak, vulnerable nature of being human as much as I hated the Adam's apple which bobbed beneath my chin. The attempt at physical perfection grew from seeds of self-disgust.

In Bamm Bamm's room, there was no telling sheet, but I did find him posing before his closet mirror.

Aside from his enormous muscles, Bamm Bamm's stretch marks caught my eye. They were a series of parallel red rips in his skin that raked from his underarms to his pectoral muscles. As testifiable marks of growth, they were the envy of the gym.

"Jesus," I muttered, repelled.

"Yeah, *wooks wike* an eagle's talons, don't it?" Bamm Bamm said, gloating.

Bamm Bamm had first started to lift weights for football. As an offensive lineman, he needed bulk and strength. But his career ended on the sidelines of Glendale Junior College, when, in front of the team, he had struck his head coach with "a forearm shiver" for reasons clear to Bamm Bamm and to no one else.

Since no college team dared have him, he'd lifted weights seriously for the next seven years. Just two years before I spoke to him, he competed in the nation's best state show, the NPC Mr. California, but finished out of the running for the heavyweight title. Nimrod had told me that Bamm Bamm had failed to diet. Bamm Bamm explained the decision of the judges as *"powitics."*

But Bamm Bamm didn't want to talk about football or body-building, he wanted to talk about war. "They've *outwawed* it, Sam," he said, shaking his head in misery. "There are no more wars, no more *Koweas* or Vietnams. That's why we have *wifting*, and this . . ." he said, opening his closet door.

Within I saw a helmet, and the rest of his armor. He had purchased it from Thornbird Arms in the San Fernando Valley. Once every few months, he left with Freewyn, a lifter from the nearby

Fanatics Gym for a weekend war regulated by The Society for Creative Anachronism.

"I fight in a *wogue spwinter gwoup*, under a duke," Bamm Bamm said, with a touch of defiance.

His last war was waged near Scottsdale, Arizona. Within spitting distance of the I-10 freeway, Bamm Bamm and a few hundred other knights from Ciad (the Southern California district) fought Adenvelt (the Arizona district) for their kingdom.

Bamm Bamm had forty "kills" that weekend, and a broken nose. Though the weapons are made of rattan, the armor is real. When a poleax struck his steel helmet, the nose guard came down and spliced his nose.

But Bamm Bamm wasn't counting on fighting for Ciad much longer. In fact, as soon as he collected the money, he planned on emigrating to Australia.

"It's a *fwontier* town, you know," he said testily. "People know what's *wight* there. They *wespect* a man for his size," he sniffed.

Muscles as merit badges and armor. God, that too seemed familiar. I who could remember every test score I'd ever received back to the second grade, yet couldn't remember half my teachers' names. I who had cynically selected every academic institution I'd attended not for its offerings but for its reputation. I'd been far less interested in an education than in documented proof of scholarly success. Even Bamm Bamm's search for war wasn't too different from my own entry into the gym. As long as we created for ourselves a rite of passage, we could instill our lives with meaning. Knights errant both, we wore our weight-lifting belts over one shoulder like baldrics, packing our own form of heat in the event of Armageddon. How much easier it made life, whether the enemy was Adenvelt or my Adam's apple or meat with more than 15 percent fat.

I wasn't at all reassured by what I had heard from Nimrod and Bamm Bamm, just saddened—about them, about me. And when I found Vinnie in his room, my self-doubts only grew.

There among the boxes of Huggies and the baby food, the cartons of steroids and the vitamins, a photographic portrait caught my eye. I hadn't seen it before. It showed a much younger and tinier Vinnie with his arms wrapped around his kid brother back in New

York. It had been taken before Vinnie found his way to the gym, that much I knew, because in every photo since then he stood before the camera as straight and stiff and grim as a soldier.

"You like photos, Sam?" Vinnie asked.

"Sure," I answered.

"Yuh don't say?" Vinnie continued, visibly excited. "You know, I've been doin' a lot of picture work, lately? Did you know that? Did you know I got acting talent?" Vinnie peered at me as if wondering whether I could be trusted. Deciding in my favor, he returned from his closet with a large professional black portfolio.

"See, I can go somewhere in this field here. Hey, you don't have to just own a gym like Raoul, or sell shit," Vinnie said, unzipping the great book and opening it.

There crouched Vinnie, fishing rod in hand, completely naked, a pastoral stage set behind him and a stream made from what looked like Saran Wrap before him. There he was in another photo, starkers once more, this time in a classroom setting, sporting an elongated dunce cap and an erection, as he serviced a bespectacled girl, who, I gathered, was the teacher in the scene. She, in turn, comforted the nether regions of a pimply faced female pupil who squatted before her.

"You know, Sam, bodybuilding presents a number of film and still opportunities," Vinnie said as I flipped through the pages.

One photo in particular caught my eye. It was a mermaid. She looked so sad, so vulnerable, that my heart went out to her.

"That's Mandy," Vinnie shouted, ripping the photo out of my hands. "Shit, does that chick have bedpan eyes or what? Sam, I really felt somethin' for her. I mean, she could suck a hubcap off a cab from twenty feet."

He looked at me suddenly with concern: "Look, Sam, don't tell Nimrod or Bamm Bamm 'bout none of this, OK? See, for now, it only pays the rent, but soon, I'll make it to higher budget things."

It didn't come as a complete surprise. From my reading of the muscle books, I knew that bodybuilding and pornography had always been inextricably intertwined. Eugene Sandow at the turn of the century posed, for cold cash and public titillation, in a glass booth and a fig leaf. His follower, Bernarr Macfadden sold photographs of his hard physique in the buff. These sold well. Those of his wife in flesh tights sold better. And, in recent history, Serge Nubret, Arnold's rival in the early seventies, had done hard-core film work in France.

As I sat beside Vinnie and drank my protein shake down to the lees (a sprinkling of lecithin granules, the yolky remains of a raw egg), I worried about my own possible future in the still and film world. I feared that complete exposure might reveal a lagging body part to the judges.

9.

THE VOCATIONAL OPPORTUNITIES

"WHO IS HE?" TENDS TO ACCOMPANY "WHAT IS HE?" AND SOMETIMES TO PRECEDE IT, AND THE CONSEQUENCES IN LIFE AS IN ART ARE COMIC OR TRAGIC, OR IN THE GREAT GREY WASTES BETWEEN.

*—PETER STANSKY
AND WILLIAM ABRAHAMS*

My mother tried. God, how she tried. Through the mail came a ceramic toothbrush rack in the shape of a muscular torso, a porcelain toilet roll holder made of bulging biceps. I was on her mind, that much was clear.

To her friends, she called me "a substance in search of a form." I wasn't really a bodybuilder, she explained, I was Baudelaire. In place of dyed green hair and revolutionary poesy, I, iron iconoclast, simpy substituted "the Walk" and the shock of drug-fed muscles. Like the long line of artists who had preceded me, I spent my days throwing bricks through stained-glass windows in my own manner.

That was her public stance, at least. In private, she fretted that I had chosen for myself a long and arduous form of suicide. My father was less charitable. He didn't give me the benefit of an aesthetic creed, however wayward. "I can feel your contempt, Son," he had written in a recent letter. "Since you first emerged crying from your mother's womb, you've always begrudged the world for its failure to measure up."

To him, I wasn't an agent provocateur or even a grotesquerie, but a derelict, plain and simple. "I understand the urge to spit," he wrote to his son, the muscle stooge, "but does it have to be facing the wind?" He had sent me but one communication since then, enclosing the heavily underlined Frost poem, "The Road Not Taken," and the University of Pennsylvania Law School application.

But if to my parents my life in bodybuilding represented the perils of free will, to my friends at Oxford the whole thing sounded Falstaffian, as if I were reveling in Southern California as some kind of anarchic Lord of Misrule. They thought the whole thing sounded sort of fun, until, that is, the photographs of my juiced-up body circulated. Then, with these bloated, billowing muscle shots in hand, they thought the whole thing kind of *sick*. The suggestive "Samuel *is* looking rather butch" progressed to the dismissive "obviously he's gone queer." Even my most loyal friend couldn't conceal his apprehension: "You have really worked a transformation of your outer self, Samuel, and I would be fascinated to know how you motivated yourself to lift weights with such diligence and faithfulness. I am curious because when, years ago, I seriously considered trying to become a concert pianist, I was unable to make myself persevere through the tedium of practice; and I tend to imagine that biceps curls and bench presses must be the finger exercises of bodybuilding."

But if iron hadn't yet reached Oxford, it had reached every other pocket of the globe. The television in our living room showed bodybuilders in commercials, in sitcoms, even in game shows. Shows like "American Gladiators" and "Roller Games" presented contestants with bulging biceps and names like "Nasty Nancy" Wilkinson and "Deadly Debbie" Van Doren. NO GAIN, NO PAIN, proclaimed billboards advertising Weightwatchers, the diet group. "Start Wheatlifting," our television commanded, displaying a muscular fist gripping a spoon freighted with shredded wheat. "Family Feud" pitted a gaggle of Gold's Gym builders against a nuclear family. Every beer advertisement seemed to have one of the diseased pumping weights in the background. And in the magazines and newspapers, the models in their underwear no longer languorously lounged *in contra posto*. Now they "stood relaxed" with sharply defined abdominal muscles and blooming pectorals. It had gone as far as the White House, where President Reagan was photographed pumping out a few bicep reps on his chrome dumbbells before a briefing. Clearly, this whole muscle thing was no longer just *my* problem.

With the obsession, came the demand. Vinnie started grossing $40,000 a year from his steroid sales. It wasn't the bodybuilders who kept his answering machine working day and night, it was the Kips and Corkys, the lawyers and bank managers and salesmen of Southern California. From Santa Monica to Cucamonga, Alhambra to San Dimas, Vinnie visited gym after gym and sold 90 percent of his goods to yuppies in tights and tank tops. Blanks or not, there was no shortage of supply, and the daily bombardments from the media, in print, television, and radio form, ensured the frenzied demand. Most of Vinnie's clients didn't realize that the drugs only worked in conjunction with training.

Vinnie wasn't my only roommate making money off the body boom. In their own way, both Bamm Bamm and Nimrod profited from their physiques. Bamm Bamm's calling was as collector for a loan shark. Overdue payments meant an appearance of Bamm Bamm at the door. And it was copious quantities of both the gym and "the juice" that kept him employed. Every few weeks, I woke at night and watched him pound past my room, his massive arms laden with spoil. Our living room became an appliance stockroom, filled with Frigidaires, microwaves, toasters, and Mr. Coffee machines. It wasn't just appliances—Bamm Bamm added to his loot diamond rings and metal mugs, silver picture frames, even leather boots.

Nimrod chose personal training. "At your home, at your office, at your gym, at your convenience!" read his embossed card. His answering machine closed with the line: "My specialty is results!" Actually, Vinnie's specialty was older women, and two or three of them a day could be counted upon to visit him in his room, to emerge light-headed and refreshed an hour later. Nimrod called it "Rolfing" and "Deep Tissue Massage." I called it something else; since then, I've known many a builder similarly equipped for aiding clients in need.

None of my bodybuilding friends worked more than a few hours a day. Anything more would have interfered with their training, their sleeping, and their eating. But work in a fashion they did— even Macon and Lamar, who pounded their beat as mall cops.

In fact, by the summer of 1987, I found myself in demand. A man hired me on sight to throw his brother into a swimming pool in front of three hundred guests on his fortieth birthday. I collected $250.00 for twenty minutes work. I did "the Walk" into photographers' studios and posed for medical calendars. The television shows "Alien Nation" and "thirtysomething" called, and, do-rag and all, I strolled before the cameras for the obligatory gym scenes.

The timing was perfect for me. After three years, I *had* to find a way of giving my lifting purpose and meaning. It had begun to dawn on me that the whole building thing might be merely a parody of labor, and I myself a well-muscled dilettante. What would Jeremy Bentham, the father of utilitarianism, think of bodybuilding? He had to be turning over in his grave. After all, the iron we lifted didn't help build a bridge or a battleship or a skyscraper. It enlarged our biceps and spread the sweep of our thighs. The labor of farmers and factory workers and longshoremen had a kind of dignity and purpose that ours didn't.

A muscle vocation was the answer to my private panic, I was sure of it. If I could get a job related to my body, then I'd feel less self-indulgent; function and form would be in better balance. But the modeling jobs and the extra work came along too infrequently. I needed something more. Lucky for me, then, that by 1987 personal trainers like Nimrod were as much in demand as cellular car phones. And doubly lucky, the supply was so small and the demand so great that no credentials were needed other than a lifter's physique.

All I lacked, Nimrod said, to start my career at Shangri-La, was the assent of Raoul, since our gym did not allow independent instruction. With his approval, I could begin to train clients immediately, though I would be placed on probationary status. I would then be given a year to successfully complete a CPR course and a standardized test for personal trainers developed for IDEA (the International Dance and Exercise Association) by the Educational Testing Service (the same folks who brought us the SAT). The regulated wage at Shangri-La was $30.00 an hour, of which the gym received a $5.00 cut.

Two years earlier, back in New York, Fowler had said to me: "Sam, do you have any idea how this will look on your resumé?"

"What? How what will look on my resumé?"

"This," Fowler said, waving his hand over my T-shirted torso.

But it was just this torso, now 'roided and juiced to the tune of 250 pounds, that I presented to Shangri-La to begin my life as a personal trainer.

I found Raoul, sunken-cheeked and shriveled, in his back office. The dark room was bathed in the green, ghostly light of his computer screen. On the desk before him was a partially nibbled rice cake and a bottle of distilled water. The office was crammed with boxes containing his mail-order catalog goods: training manuals, car shades, personalized weight-lifting belts, signature protein powders, his own line of clothes, posters, place mats, key chains, 8 × 10 autographed glossies. Raoul had the goods, but for whatever reason, America wasn't biting.

"My products, they won't move," he moaned.

His investors were irate. Raoul hadn't trained in months, he was too preoccupied with his losses. And it showed—behind his desk, he looked tinier than a Tibetan Sherpa. He barely seemed to hear me when I asked his permission to train clients, but he gave me the nod.

I left him with his head bowed before the unopened copies of *Esquire, GQ,* and *Business Week* arranged precisely on his desk. Still working on his overall presentation, I gathered. It all made sense somehow, Raoul and bodybuilding.

The next morning, I penciled in my hours at the trainers' log book at Tara's front desk. Not long after, I heard her call my name on the gym's PA system. "Attention Sam, your 10:30 is here."

So began my life as a personal trainer. I met my first client at the Trainer's Table in the foyer and gave him the company line as I took a seat: "Good morning, it's a great day at Shangri-La Fitness Training Center!" I heard myself roar. "My name is Sam, and how may I help you?"

And help them I did. During "the initial consultation" I guided my new clients through the maze of personal information I needed in order to "design" their program. Before prescribing my training recommendations, I jotted down their exercise history, their medical history, and, as calmly as possible, any emergency phone numbers and next of kin.

I took their blood pressure, I measured their pulse, I established their "target heart rate," their "desired workload," all the while explaining the logic and simplicity of the endeavor. To change your appearance, I said, merely reduce the quantity of fat in your diet while simultaneously increasing the fat-burning activity in your exercise. Fat-burning activity included the Lifecycle (a gussied up stationary bicycle), the treadmill, high-speed circuit training, or aerobics classes like Bodysculpt, Motion Explosion, Cardiofunk, and Power Aerobics, all Shangri-La specialties.

No consultation was complete without recourse to my metal calipers. The hydrostatic method is the most accurate means to estimate body fat, lowering clients like livestock into a pool of water and noting water displacement. But Shangri-La didn't have a pool for the hydrostatic method, nor did we have electrical-stimulation equipment, so we used our metal calipers. Raoul handed me an oversized pair that looked like something out of a horror film, and these I plied in so-called "skinfold measurements," as my manual said, "for field assessment of body composition."

As Raoul had done with me a year earlier, I tugged the flesh between thumb and forefinger at certain target sites. For men, the sites included (1) the chest ("halfway between the nipple and the shoulder crease"); (2) the axilla ("a line bisecting the armpit and hip at a level equal to the xiphoid process"); (3) the triceps; (4) the subscapula ("diagonal fold just under the bottom angle of the scapula; halfway between the spine and the side of the body"); (5) the suprailiac ("just above the iliac crest; slightly anterior to the middle of the side"); and (6) the thigh ("halfway between the greater trochanter and the patella").

For women, the chest was not to be pinched, though everything else was. The company manual had words of wisdom for testing female clients: "In some cases when measuring a member of the opposite sex, you may want to use a witness."

According to my company chart, the "ideal" body-fat percentage for men was 15, the Southern California average 22, the U.S. average 26. For women, the "ideal" was 22, the Southern California average 28–30, and the U.S. average 36.

Florists, bouncers, barmen, hairstylists, I taught them all how to heave and hoist iron and how to alter their appearance. I stood vigil in my red company-issue polo shirt (with the word TRAINER emblazoned in yellow on the back) while they walked or ran on the treadmill or pedaled on the Lifecycle. Most of my clients I saw three times per week, one hour per session. Moët I saw six days a week.

I met her husband first. "Oh, hi! My name's Evan!" he said, interrupting my workout. "I've been done by Bruce—Bruce Weber." He raised his eyebrows expectantly and, at my lack of response, rolled his eyes. "The photographer," he moaned, exasperated.

"I don't understand," I said. "Do you need a trainer?"

"God no! It's not me!" Evan blurted out. "I'm a *model*. No, it's my main squeeze, Moët."

The next day, Moët sat beside me for her consultation. I took down the relevant information.

"Last name?" I asked.

"Just Moët," she chirped, "as in Sting or Cher."

Actually, it was Moët as in champagne. She'd read about Margaux Hemingway in *People* Magazine, thought the name classy, and spoke to her lawyer the same day. Goodbye Dulcie. Hello Moët.

A chin cleft, a buttock and tummy tuck through liposuction, cheekbone implants, a nose job—Moët was a firm believer in modern science. But it was her boob job that was most noticeable. The doctor had left her with a pair so massive that she needed three bras at once for support. She seemed in danger of collapsing forward from the weight at any given moment.

As much as the gym rats couldn't avoid gawking at them, Moët couldn't get them off of her mind. She had a mania concerning her breasts. All conversation, eventually, returned to them.

As we trained, my standard query "Are you all right?" became, in her ears, "Are they all right?"

"I think they're better now, thanks. My doctor told me the skin would retract around them after the operation, and I'd feel corsetted, but I didn't expect them to be this tight."

It wasn't always her breasts: "I went in for lip augmentation last week, you know," she said. "See, the doctor harvests fat from my thigh and injects it into my lips. Some people use bovine collagen, but it's so much more natural to use your own fat, don't you think?"

"Oh yes!" I said, enthusiastically. "Try to keep 'continuous tension' on your triceps."

"Oh right . . . well, it's made a world of difference, Sam. See, they're much fuller now. I go twice a year, just for a touch-up. I really love this soft pout. I mean, it's a really good look."

"Your breasts?" I asked, handing her a chrome dumbbell for her superset.

"No, silly, my lips," she responded, pumping out more reps.

"How does your husband like it?" I asked.

"Evan? Are you kidding? At cocktail parties, in movie lines, wherever we go, you should see the rubberneckers!

"Oh, who is that?" Moët moaned, spotting what she called a "GLD" (or Good Looking Dude) by the squat machine. "Sam, I think I just stopped *breathing!* And look, my nipples are getting hard, and gosh, look how they're sweating."

For six straight months, I trained her six days a week. Only once did she need to take time off, for the hospital as it happened. "Remember, Sam," she told me. "I'm going in for surgery next week."

She paused on the conveyer belt of the treadmill. "I'm finally having those two ribs near the bottom removed. It will really make my waist look different. You know, you don't live your dreams, you die."

"What is that, Nietzsche?" I asked, checking her target heart rate.

"No, *Flashdance,*" she said, picking up her pace on the road to nowhere.

I nodded wearily, adjusted the speed of the treadmill and murmured "make haste slowly." At least, I think it was "make haste slowly." Then again, it might have been, "you work hard, good things will happen," or "be here now," or "no guts, no glory," or "she who dares, wins," or "bigger's better," or a host of other muscle clichés.

I retreated into the world of iron platitudes because the few times I fell out of character, the result was invariably an absurd misconnection, a dialogue of the deaf, which sent me scurrying back for cover.

Such was the case with my 9:30, Brock. He spent his sixty minutes on the stationary bicycle, and paid me $30.00 an hour to talk to him. One day, he happened to ask me about my relatives. I started with my uncle. While Brock pedaled and puffed, I spoke.

"More than anything," I said, "he was a man of principle. During the 1950s, he taught at Berkeley, and refused to sign the document stating he was not a Communist. They fired him for it."

"Really? it takes a lot of integrity to do that," Brock said, excited. "That is really admirable. I've got a client like that. His name is Jim Thurnbull, owns the biggest tire factory in the U.S., Thurnbull Tires, you've heard of it, right? Anyway, he's trying to find the best bidder for his company. Well, the Nips, they're offering him the most money, but you know what? He'd rather sell to an American. Men like Thurnbull and your uncle, they make America great!"

There was no escape, no matter how I tried. When I fled my clients, things only got worse. Once, after the usual session with Moët (or was it Gino, or Melissa, or Steve, or Trixie?), I padded to the locker room, collapsed on a wooden stool, and held my head in my hands.

"Don't be such a sissy, son!" I heard someone shout over by the sink. "This is strength juice!"

It was Macon, and as I walked onto the tiles, I saw him hovering over the kneeling Lamar. Together, they looked like Abraham and a muscle-bound Isaac. In one upraised hand, Macon sported a syringe. Lamar, his Mohawked head bowed, offered his enormous white ass to his father.

"Just supplementing, Sam, just supplementing," Macon whispered to me with a wink. "Time for Lamar's feeding, if you know what I mean. . . ." He hugged his son with one arm before striking him with the syringe.

Despite the jolt of the needle, Lamar looked up at his father in tenderness. Together, they formed a loving lifting diptych, but I'd barely survived that first treacly night back at the Maverick, and this was just too much.

Between my clients and my own workouts, I was now spending twelve hours a day in the gym. It wasn't my four daily hours of workouts that bothered me. It was the eight hours of instruction or roaming the floor, clipboard and calipers in hand, eight hours of observing my clients and fellow gym members, eight hours in which I saw nothing but iron casualties. The place harbored multitudes of them—cleft palates, speech impediments, club feet, PWC's (People

With Causes: militant vegetarians, animal rights activists, Christers).
Shangri-La, like the Y before it, was a breeding ground for the inept,
the inane, and, when it came down to it, the homeless.

And it was beginning to dawn on me that I was one of them.
How different was the Arnold I kept in my mind from the tattered
portrait of Bill Pearl painted on black velvet in an imitation wood
frame that Leonard carted with him in the gym and out? Watching
Leonard work out, accompanied by the portrait, was amusing.
Watching him eat at a table for two, the portrait seated across from
him, was more disturbing. How different was I from Hector (née
Hortense), who played not rock music on his Walkman but "Crackling Fire," from the "Sound of Nature Relaxation Tape Collection."
Both of us were desperate for reassurance. I used iron and the gym,
he used the comforting sounds of the hearth. And the stutterers,
how different was I from them? They kept silent because they had to;
my aphasia was strictly voluntary. The gym was a haven for us all.

No wonder I was feeling depressed, I told myself. The answer,
I thought, might be "at home" clients, not the kind Nimrod penetrated and probed in his bedroom, but the kind who would pay me
$50.00 per hour to oversee their training in their houses or garages.
I wouldn't have to pay a kickback to Raoul; I would make twice as
much money as at the gym. I could use the gym only for my own
workouts.

With Nimrod's referrals and a stack of my own references, I was
in business. My first clients were Seymour Slatkin, the attorney,
and his wife Sheila. I trained them in their Spanish hacienda off
Orange Grove Boulevard in Pasadena every other morning. They
had transformed the central courtyard with its climbing bougain-
villaea and pocket arches into an open-air weight room.

It was the forty-five-year-old Seymour, plump and hung over,
who'd greet me first. As soon as we reached the courtyard and he
grabbed a weight, he'd begin his dramatic monologue.

"He felt the raw power surging through his body," he'd start
with a whisper, raising his voice as the reps continued. "He snapped
the man's neck like a breadstick and left him on the ground. Human
detritus! Food for flies!"

And while Seymour was off in his own world, his wife shuffled out of the breakfast room in her slippers, sweats, and hair curlers to join us for her abdominal exercises. Between sets, she whispered in my ear: "Yesterday afternoon, numbnuts over there unplugged the power on my computer while he was vacuuming the floor. Lost the whole file, the bastard."

We both looked over at Seymour. Communing with iron, he didn't notice a thing. He couldn't possibly hear her above his epic recital: "The Cajun common folk paddled from bayous beyond to catch a glimpse of Mister Man. He was big all right, but no bigger than a beer truck and with muscles to match. When he shook the beef of his bicep, it sounded like rolling thunder."

Exasperated, Sheila said, "I don't know why he does this. He never does it when he's not pumping iron, you know."

Seymour countered when he had me alone. He pointed at Sheila squatting in the corner. "At this stage, what can she do? She's lost her looks, don't you think? Hell, I'd rather screw my own mother-in-law. Hamburger instead of fish sticks—what's the difference? It's all fast food anyway. Sure you can't come in and join us for a protein shake after the workout, Sam?"

As a way of escape from all that—the gym clients, the home clients, the whole mess—I retreated to my own workouts. Full retreat meant training by myself. Much as I learned from Vinnie, his lifting was too much like a Vegas lounge act. He demanded an audience to pull him through, and I knew I spent too much time and energy helping him with his visualization principles, his ammonia, his walk, and his talk for my own good. To Vinnie, as to so many other bodybuilders, lifting was a team sport, so long as he was the team and his training partner provided the support.

But I loved iron not for its offering of a community, but for its promise of solitude, for the chance to escape from everyone and everything. So, as gently as possible, I disengaged myself from Vinnie in the gym, and bought my own Walkman. And despite his mumbling "the student has overtaken the professor," I knew that he was secretly relieved. For a solid year, my workouts had been driving him into the ground.

Without a training partner, I found I could work that much harder. As long as I drove myself mercilessly through another sweating, bleeding, training session, I didn't think about my clients, the other gym members, my roommates, better still, I never thought about myself. I blotted everything else out and, twice a day, met the demands of three on, one off training.

Only occasionally did I stray from the endless cycle to wander the foreign land of Muscle Confusion. This was a technique I used to shock my muscles into growth by forcing them to encounter something new: dumbbell bench presses instead of barbell bench presses, say, or squats first on leg day instead of the warm-up of leg extensions.

"Adapt, adapt," I kept saying to myself, as my muscles ballooned in response to these variant exercises. As soon as I reached another plateau and found it difficult to get a pump, I tried something else: supersetting the bench with dips, leg extensions with squats. I kept my body guessing, but most of all, I kept pounding and I kept pressing.

"Give it some time, you're overtraining," all of my iron friends said when they witnessed my mad workouts.

I met their muscle clichés with my own: "There is no such thing as overtraining, only weak minds," I said, stealing the line from The Barbarian Brothers (twin lifters regularly seen in the pages of the magazines). I knew the answer couldn't be merely time, because my Shangri-La friends had all put in their ten years, like Mousie and Sweepea back in New York, yet they were still years away from competing against the best. Arnold had made himself into Mr. Universe in five years. I had already done four—time enough, I thought.

The answer couldn't be just steroids either, though they were part of it. Nor could everything be attributed to genetics, there were too many exceptions, too many bodybuilders like Franco Columbu who had succeeded despite enormous handicaps. A two-time Mr. Olympia, he had overcome bowlegs and the gnarled, stumpy frame of a garden gnome. No, the answer had to be simpler: never missing a workout, exercising with intensity, feeling every movement. Bodybuilders aren't born, but made.

As I pursued my quest, I found that even had I been willing, no one would have trained with me.

"Doing legs today?" I'd occasionally ask Moses or Lamar or Nimrod.

In return, I'd get a nervous look. "No man, chest," was the wary reply.

If it was chest day for me, it would be leg day for them. It wasn't personal, it was simply survival. The only lifter capable of surviving my workouts was me. Just like back at the New York Y, no one else was so desperate to lose consciousness, if only for two hours. No one else was so saddened or disappointed or terrified by reality to need such an anodyne.

In the gym, I out-Vinnied even Vinnie in muscle intensity, in muscle isolation, in muscle integrity. "OH JOY!" I screamed as soon as I felt the cold iron dumbbell in my hand. Safe once more. And it worked—the reps, the sets, the muscles kept *everyone* at bay. Not just the muggers and street thugs, but friends and family, even dates.

Especially dates. Muscle isolation didn't permit it. Nimrod, on a cash and carry basis, counted on his clients for occasional favors and Vinnie could always rely on his AA meetings for the nameless sexual encounters these occasions of sobriety provided, but I hadn't had a date since I moved to California.

The prospect of dating terrified me. It ran counter to my life's work, bodybuilding. To date meant to admit frailty, to acknowledge the fact that I was less than complete. Nimrod, Bamm Bamm, Vinnie, Lamar, none of us had meaningful relationships with anything other than iron. Such was the case, anyway, until Nimrod told me of G-spot's feelings.

"She has a serious jones for you, Big Man," he said.

Thus ensued a parody of a date, complete with flowers, wine and muscle-wooing. At 1404 Delacey, I dimmed the lights, smoothed the sofa, and put an album on the stereo (Nimrod's posing music, it so happened). My three roommates aided the cause by decamping to a Schwarzenegger movie.

It wasn't long before the burly G-spot parked her pickup on the lawn and presented me with photographs from her competition album. I hardly recognized her in these "before" shots, in which she chaired her high school debate team and played horseshoes with her family. The girl in these photographs was slender, attractive, a veritable gamine.

But that was long ago; the woman in my arms was someone else. As G-spot put it with her winning smile and her foghorn voice, "I've fucking reversed the course of nature."

Menarche had halted with the introduction of steroids to her system. The coarse facial hair and acne started soon after. To counteract the sweat, she used spritz; to counteract the muscles, makeup. In fact, on the sofa, in my arms, G-spot looked like she'd strayed into mommy's makeup cabinet. She wore more rouge, lipstick, and powder than a Regent Street bawd.

Between the two of us, there was close to five hundred pounds on that sofa, and when our grappling session began, you could practically hear the clink and groan of armor. There was barely room for our lips to meet above our swollen, pumped up chests. When, finally, I reached below her gold dumbbell pendant for her breast, I found it harder than my own.

I couldn't go through with it that night. Neither could she. Secretly, we were both content. Our moats and drawbridges had held after all.

I was a bodybuilder, all right, inside and out. Now, thanks to the juice, I had in abundance the thickness and muscle maturity I had once lacked. No one delivered more muscle lines with more authority (if not conviction) than I did. No one had fewer dates. I had become my own bunker.

By May of 1988, I weighed 257 pounds. My neck measured 19 inches. It was wider than my head. My arms measured 18 inches cold (without the added bloat of the pump), my calves 17½. I had a 52-inch chest, a 36-inch waist, and 29-inch thighs. God knows, I looked the part. The only thing remaining to complete the persona was competition.

I viewed it as nothing more than what I'd been doing in an informal manner in the gym for so long. I was just increasing the level of competition, I reasoned to myself, seeking better opponents. But the truth was, I prayed that with a title I'd feel less constricted, less fraudulent, comfortable for more than my four hours of training every day. Everything else in the muscle world, I'd tried. Only a trophy remained to confirm my new identity.

10.

THE NINTH ANNUAL ROSE CITY BENCH-PRESS EXTRAVAGANZA

IF SOMEONE MADE THE SLIGHTEST REMARK OR GAVE ME TROUBLE, I WOULD HIT THEM OVER THE HEAD.

—ARNOLD SCHWARZENEGGER

Thus it was that in June of 1988 I silently took Vinnie's arm and led him toward the bulletin board on the gym wall. The cork surface was filled with notices and cards advertising discount massages, vitamin and supplement sales, rowing-machine deals, and at-home training sessions.

Vinnie's eyes skimmed over these to focus on three flyers. One heralded an upcoming strength event, the other two bodybuilding contests.

"Boom, boom, boom," I said.

Vinnie looked back at me and smiled. "In the final arena, there will be no judges, Sam, only witnesses to your greatness!" he shouted, collaring me with one arm and flourishing an upraised fist with the other.

I had six weeks until the Ninth Annual Rose City Bench-Press Extravaganza, then seven weeks more until Mr. San Gabriel Valley, after that, a week until Mr. Golden Valley. Scheduled for July thirtieth, the first show was a powerlifting contest, not a bodybuilding competition. There would be no posing or flexing, just pushing weight against gravity. As I had told my publishing friends two years earlier back in New York, in a "full power meet," the athlete performs three attempts at each of the three different lifts: the squat, the bench press, and the deadlift over the course of one full day.

But the Ninth Annual Rose City Bench-Press Extravaganza eschewed the squat and the deadlift in favor of the bench press—and for a reason. Among powerlifters, the bench press is the definable you, the real you. "What's your bench?" is the classic greeting among powerlifters, as indicative of a man's worth as "Where did you go to college?" among the flannel-trousered crowd or "What do you make per year?" where polyester rules.

To the scorn of powerlifters, bodybuilders invariably give as their response the poundage they bounce. But since most lifters can bounce at least 50 more pounds than they can pause, it is not an appropriate answer. The pause is the moment, lasting as long as one full second when the bar meets your chest and simply rests there. Once the judge at the bench press sees that the bar has come to a full stop, he'll clap, signaling the lifter to begin the push upwards.

Twice a week, for the last four years, I had spent my bench sessions deliriously bouncing the steel bar off my chest, using my rib cage and gut as a primitive trampoline. My ego demanded the extra weight that poor form permitted. Now, finally, I had this powerlifting competition to tell me just who and what I was.

One twenty-three, 352. Those were the vital statistics of Hero Isagawa, Japanese expatriate and world-class powerlifter who trained at Shangri-La. He competes in the 123-pound class, and holds the current world bench-press record, a whopping 352 pounds, which he set at the International Powerlifting Federation World Championships in Australia in 1988.

With Hero as my guide, I learned to pause. But the bench press wasn't as simple as pausing. There was also the explosion to master— the moment the bencher ends his pause and fuels all his energy for the upward burst of the bar. The next step was learning "the initial phase of lockout." The first 10 inches off the chest, the explosion, are murder. But once you have pushed the bar past that point, you reach "the initial phase of lockout," at which, comparatively, it's smooth sailing. According to powerlifting physics, the last 12 inches of the movement, the simple locking out, is half as difficult as the first 12 for a man with the wingspan of an albatross, like me.

But the real key to the bench, Hero said, lies in overcoming the fear of heavy poundages. I'd heard all about bench-press injuries as far back as Austin in the New York Y. Ripped pectorals, separated shoulders, missing teeth, anything could happen from wayward bars and awkward form, said some. But Hero scoffed at my iron anecdotes. He told me that if these sources were to be trusted, then

Arnold's constant companion wasn't Maria Shriver, but a kidney dialysis machine; then professional bodybuilder Rich Gaspari collapsed once monthly from excessive steroid intake; then half the world was caught in the grip of a "'roid rage." It was all just muscle malarkey, Hero said.

Instead of fearing what could happen to me, why not concentrate on what I could make happen? he asked. Misty eyed, he told me of the men with "the attitudes fantastic," the drooling and hysterical powerlifters, who once a year convened in Hawaii for the Budweiser World Record Breakers and hoisted weights previously thought untenable.

At this Hawaiian strength-fest, Ted Arcidi had bench pressed 705 pounds; Fred Hatfield, also known as Dr. Squat, had been the first to officially squat over a thousand pounds. Here the superheavyweights (those weighing over 275 pounds) were so huge, they had to use a meat scale instead of a Medco at the weigh-in. Here, superheavyweights (some of them weighing as much as four hundred pounds themselves) routinely broke the 2,000 total barrier (a powerlifter's meet total equals his best squat, plus best bench, plus best deadlift of that day). For the superheavies, this routinely meant squatting over eight hundred pounds, benching around six hundred, and deadlifting a good eight hundred as well.

Hero regaled me with these tales while I took a sabbatical from "Intensity or Insanity" training. I had to. Powerlifters and bodybuilders train in a most dissimilar fashion. Powerlifters do not profit from smooth, endless repetitions. The 12 to 15 reps per set with lighter weights that had worked so well for shaping were now a distinct disadvantage. Four to 5 reps of much higher weight and far fewer sets were the powerlifting norm. And in between these sets were the rest periods, not the 60 seconds that I practiced as a bodybuilder, but 10 to 15 minutes, simulating powerlifting competitions where a bevy of competitors have to lift in between your attempts. Out with "continuous tension," in with full muscle recovery.

To powerlifters, bodybuilders are a fraud, all muscles but no real strength. The bodybuilder's endless reps are not recognized as a strength by powerlifters, anymore than a sprinter recognizes the merits of a marathoner. And bodybuilders reserve similar scorn for powerlifters, whose 1-rep strength they admire, but whose physiques, without veins or definition, they abjure.

Which made it all the odder to my bodybuilding friends that I was entering a powerlifting meet. As the two sports have evolved, no one has ever combined expertise in both. The extremism of each training style necessitates choosing one or the other. But I couldn't do just the bodybuilding shows. I had to prove to myself, if to no one else, that my muscles weren't simply decorative.

As the flyer noted, there were five different divisions in the bench-press competition: Masters (of which there were two divisions, ages 40–46 and 47–53); Open (male lifters who have competed in four or more meets); Novice (male lifters aged 20 and above who have competed in three meets or less); Women (all ages, all weight classes); and Teenage (male lifters ages 14–19).

Hero advised me to enter the contest as a novice at 243 pounds, one pound up from the 242-pound-weight-class limit. This was perfect. Although I weighed 257, I had to diet anyway for my bodybuilding contests, and if I could get down to 243 by July thirtieth, it would make it easier to reach 230 and 6 percent body fat for the physique shows in late September.

Hero's counsel, though, had nothing to do with bodybuilding and everything to do with winning a bench-press trophy. As he pointed out, weighing 243 the day of the contest would put me in the 275-pound-weight class, where the competition in minor shows is notoriously weak.

As proof, he brought out his back issues of *Powerlifting USA*. I flipped past the pages advertising "Deadlift Shoes," "Super Chalk," *Ernie's Workout Log Book*, and special squat suits "guaranteed against crotch blow-out." I headed for the final pages and the minuscule print of results from regional competitions over the past six months. Sure enough, Hero was right. The results were consistent: Whether it was the Biggest Bench on the Beach (Des Moines, IA), the 5th New London Open Bench Press (New London, CT), the 2nd Illinois Valley Bench Press (Peru, IL), the Bench-A-Mania (Stanardsville, VA), the 5th Annual Bayou Classic (Monroe, LA), the 275-pound-class lifters always benched less than those in the 181, 198, and 220 classes.

Those lighter classes featured men like the five foot three inch, 181-pound Mike Bridges, with barrel chests and truncated arms—the perfect build for benching. At six foot four, I would be at a distinct disadvantage. But I wouldn't have to compete against them. If everything went according to plan, I probably wouldn't have to compete against anyone, because there was a paucity of competitors in the 275-pound class in the novice division around the country. If I could just make my opening lift, I'd probably win a trophy; the flyer announced first, second, and third place trophies for *every* weight class.

One thing I didn't have to worry about for my strength contest (or the bodybuilding contests to follow) was drug detection. The flyers for these meets did not include the "natural" or "drug-free" warnings that occasionally accompanied the notice of a show. This omission was a signal to all competitors that there would not be a polygraph or urinalysis test on the day of the competition.

But only the credulous public buys the distinction between "drug-free" and drugged. All strength athletes, whether powerlifters, bodybuilders or Olympic weight lifters, know that the tests are laughably flawed. The brilliant minds of science may be coming up with the tests, but they are also helping athletes defeat their purpose. When Ziegler first began perfecting steroids for strength athletes back in '58, he was acting in the interest of national prestige (read nationalist paranoia). The Soviet weight-lifting team was said to be experimenting with testosterone. If we didn't catch up to them, we would be disgraced.

Generated in this spirit, the steroid war has never pitted athletes against scientists, but scientists against scientists. The real race isn't out on the track or in the gym, but in the labs. Doctors are, after all, human, and as susceptible to Olympic medal tally obsession as the man at home in front of his television set in Manhattan or Minsk.

And as the steroid war has moved to the eighties, for every scientist who improves the drug test to detect chemical masking agents (like probenicid), there's another scientist who discovers a new masking agent (like Azubromaron, Anturane, or Carinamide) to prevent detection. Or there's a scientist who designs a new strength drug altogether, like human growth hormone, which is, to date, undetectable. As Dan Duchaine, author of the *Underground Steroid Handbook*, writes in *Modern Bodybuilding*, "the drug test, even at the IOC (International Olympic Committee) level, is failed primarily by uninformed athletes."

To ensure my strength, I "stacked" my drugs for the seven weeks before the contest, no longer relying on just my usual blend of testosterone cypionate, Anavar, and Deca (2 ccs, 70 pills, and 4 ccs per week, respectively) but 3 ccs per week of Equipoise as well. Vinnie bought a 30-cc vial of this horse drug from a veterinarian who worked at Santa Anita Race Track. On the label were illustrations of bulls, horses, dogs, and pigs. According to Vinnie, it worked as a muscle and strength builder for humans, too.

"Look, Sam, you think they gonna mistreat five million dollar thoroughbreds?" Vinnie first asked me when I questioned him on Equipoise. To Vinnie, the argument was simple. Their "net worth" far exceeded mine.

Since I didn't have to worry about my drug program, I worried about my Inzer Blast Shirt. Actually, it belonged to Lamar, but he gave it to me when he heard that I was soon to compete. Lamar and his father wanted to lend me The Outlaw, which was, as Macon confided "the God damn Rolls Royce of lifting suits," but it was designed specifically for squatting and deadlifting, which wouldn't help me much in a bench-press contest.

The Inzer Blast Shirt's whole raison d'être was benching. It guaranteed the user an increase of 20 to 35 pounds on his personal best. This sounded wonderful—it might just push me over the 400-pound barrier, since 385 was my personal best.

All shiny red nylon and rigid, it looked harmless enough in Lamar's hands. But from the very beginning, when Lamar and Macon took turns stretching it over my torso in the locker room, we encountered difficulty. It took 5 full minutes to tug and draw the material over my head. I patiently stood with my arms raised to the sky as the boys broke into a sweat just rolling it down my chest and stomach. Macon had to prop his foot against my ass to get enough leverage to pull the constricting fabric down my back.

The tighter it was, the better, they said. It would give me a feeling of security. It would prevent an injury. It would keep my arms in the benching groove. All the world champions wore them, Hero included. It was tight, all right, so tight that the fabric propelled my arms forward. I looked like a sleepwalker as I waddled to take my place on the bench. But this was precisely how the shirt was supposed to work. "Designed to aid and support your bench press throughout the entire range of motion," the shirt's main function was to *limit* that range of motion. I couldn't eat or bowl or use the toilet wearing the Inzer Blast Shirt, but by God I could bench.

Macon warned me that I might experience a minor degree of discomfort as he lowered the bar to my grasp. Lamar often did on the first set, he said. But I screamed in pain when the bar fell to my chest. I could actually feel my skin tearing underneath my armpits. Lamar was delighted. That proved it. A perfect fit, he said.

At the end of the workout, it wasn't much better, and when Lamar and Macon rolled the shirt off me and I looked in the mirror, I saw that my upper body was a collection of bruises and raw, open sores. It had done the trick, though, increasing my bench press to 405 pounds, with a lengthy pause, no less. Lamar let me borrow it for the duration. In return, I bought Cuddles some nutritionally sound biscuits.

Everything was going to plan—the Inzer Blast Shirt, the actual lifting, the diet, the mental mood. All were in place. If I could just nail 405 pounds in the contest, I was sure I would not only win my weight class, but raise a number of eyebrows as well.

Was I ready? Well, I ripped the safety brake of Vinnie's Luv right out of its socket when I pulled up to the digs that afternoon. At Shangri-La, 12 hours before the meet, I weighed in at 243. But that night, there was trouble. As I lay in bed, I had difficulty breathing. Was it the Equipoise? In a last dash for greatness, I had thrown caution to the wind and had been secretly injecting myself with 4 ccs of the stuff per week. Since food seemed to flow through me unimpeded, multiple injections were the only way I could maintain enough bodyweight to enter the contest in the 275-pound category.

It wasn't my asthma that bothered me, though. It was my heart. It pounded uncontrollably, a resting 120 beats per minute, in fact. It might well have been the testosterone too, since I had also upped that dosage to 4 ccs per week. Or it could have been simply nerves. *Powerlifting USA* displayed exceedingly large men with abnormally low brows. In fact, the promoter of tomorrow's meet was also the promoter of the Budweiser World Record Breakers in Hawaii. Tomorrow's contest featured $1,400 in cash prizes. Men who actually made their living at this might be there. No, I didn't get a wink of sleep that night. I had just finished my breakfast when Vinnie came knocking the morning of the contest.

"Time to kick ass and take names, Big Man," he charged, with thin-lipped severity.

Outside the Y, the line of powerlifters in transit, all clad in sweatsuits advertising their gyms, perked me up. There were representatives from each of the five different divisions, but none of them looked big enough to be in my weight class. Everything was going according to plan. As Vinnie left me to tour the competition room, I joined the group of strength specialists and sat with them in the building's lobby.

I spotted two empty seats next to a human light bulb. He had a great barrel chest and sparrow stalks for legs (Sweepea back in New York would have known him for what he was—a bar body). His black face bore blue tattooes, a series of tears running down one cheek. It was difficult to tell from his lopsided body, but I estimated he was in the 220-pound class. I sat down beside him, but he didn't turn his head.

"What's up?" I asked, and then the more pertinent question: "By the way, what weight class are you in?"

Slowly, keeping his eyes fixed dead ahead, he spoke.

"The name's Titanium."

"Well, the pleasure's mine," I said. "You aren't in the 275's are you, Ty?"

"I said the name's *Titanium!*" he repeated with increasing volume.

Right. Don't talk, just let him visualize. While he ground his teeth beside me, I watched as the contestants filed through the door, from the shuffling, blue-haired geriatrics of the Masters Division to the gum-smacking, preening teens.

To my right, an elbow nudged me.

"How's it hanging?" the man said. "I'm Francis, but my friends call me Turbo." He was a Master, around fifty years old, with glasses and a paunch. His tank top said POWERLIFTERS: STRONG ENOUGH TO BEAR THE STRAIN, MAN ENOUGH TO TAKE THE PAIN.

"Just fine, how are you?" I said.

"Great. Great. The Synthroid is really working, so's the Halotestin and the Test," he said, speaking of his drug program. "Only the strong survive," he said, with a reassuring smile.

Turbo nudged me again, "Look! There's Chip Taylor—123. Open. His Schwartz is really impressive!"

Right. The Schwartz Formula. Hero had told me all about this. Invented by Lyle A. Schwartz, powerlifting enthusiast and professor of Materials Science and Engineering at Northwestern University, it is a judging system in which each lifter is assigned a numerical coefficient according to body weight. At the conclusion of the contest, all lifters are graded by multiplying their coefficient with their total lifts. The system enables, say, a 123-pound man who benches 350, to defeat a 242-pound man who benches 500.

But worrying about my Schwartz would get me nowhere. I carried far too much body weight to score well by this system. I just needed to make my first lift, my opener, and I'd win a trophy, I reminded myself.

Gus, the promoter of the meet, strode through the door. He had more muscles than Lamar, more stretch marks than Bamm Bamm. A decade of 900-pound squats, 800-pound deadlifts, and 500-pound bench presses had not gone without effect. He had played the role of "Buzzsaw" in the Schwarzenegger movie *The Running Man*.

As the last of the competitors filed in, Gus went over the official meet rules. There would be judges stationed around the bench press to apprehend cheaters, he said, and each judge would be supplied with green and red paddles. Only legal lifts would merit green paddles. The bar must come down evenly and pause at the chest.

At the sound of the clap from the head judge, the bar would be pressed upwards evenly without one side of it moving at a higher angle due to a stronger arm or shoulder until the arms locked out. But that wasn't all. Each contestant would be required to keep his feet sturdily on the floor during the lift and his bottom in continuous contact with the bench. Chalk, wrist wraps, the Inzer Blast shirt and unlimited inhalation of ammonia were legal, as in all regulation powerlifting meets.

He then passed out to each of us one complimentary program of the event itself, filled with advertisements and notes of sponsorship. Budweiser's Natural Light presented the competition, but Inzer Advance Designs ("We Make Power Gear A Science") sponsored it. I flipped through the pages advertising linear leg sleds and deluxe T-Bar Rows until I spotted the list of contestants. There were three women, at 105, 123, and 165 pounds. The men's classes began at 123 pounds, and proceeded upwards, through 132, 148, 165, 181, 198, 220, 242 to, finally, 275. I found my name—the only entrant, as expected, in the 275-pound-weight class. It was too good to be true.

Until the weigh-in, that is. There in the bowels of the Y, right by the lockers and the heater and the exposed wiring, I stepped on the Medco three separate times, and on each occasion, the bar indicated I weighed 241 pounds, one pound under the 242 limit. I couldn't believe it. I was 2 pounds off.

I had not succeeded. I would not be unopposed. There were at least two competitors who were fifteen pounds less than me, but were still above 220, and thus in my 242-pound-weight class. And though both were officially novices, they were also experienced powerlifters.

I put my sweat clothes back on and started the long trudge up the stairs to the basketball court, the sight of the actual extravaganza. I hadn't even lifted a weight yet, and already something had gone wrong. And it could get a hell of a lot worse. What if I could not make my opening lift? As powerlifters say, I would "bomb." Once you state your opening lift, you can't go lower for the next two attempts. To botch all three attempts would mean to fail even to

finish third in a weight class in which there were only three contestants. Nothing could be more humiliating.

As I neared the entrance, the noise of the crowd grew louder
and louder. At the last step, I peered out onto the court. The seats
were arranged in a horseshoe formation around the bench, and every
seat was filled. Past the heads of some of the standing spectators,
I could just make out the wooden platform, raised to the level of 4
feet. Upon the regal red rug that covered the dais, lay the majestic
steel and leather bench press.

I saw Macon, Moses, Vinnie, Lamar, and, poking out from the
Gold's Gym bag on Lamar's lap, even Cuddles in the packed audience. My stomach heaved. I tried to quell the dyspepsia with a
fistful of BIG Chewables and a multivitamin pack from my Gold's
Gym bag, but, without water, they were as difficult to get down as
gravel.

Holding on to the frame of the door for support, I caught sight
of a long table to one side of the platform, with seats for the judges.
Judges and an audience. I was on trial. If I could just nail 405 pounds
on the bench press, there would be a reprieve. The other contestants
in my weight class wouldn't matter. Four hundred and five was
respectability, actually impressive for a first-time contestant. At
least, that's what I told myself, as I emerged from the stairwell and
did "the Walk" over to the warm-up room.

The practice pit was sorely inadequate for our needs. It was
humid and steaming and almost pitch-black. During my stretching
exercises, I saw that an ugly black-white situation had developed.
The minority competitors, clearly in the majority here, had opted
to confiscate the sole practice bench press and reserve it exclusively
for members of their own race. The usual majority, here a muttering
minority, warmed up as best they could on inferior cables and
dumbbells, cursing the situation—but not very loudly.

For a few minutes, I tried the cables as well. But it was impossible.
I couldn't get limber. If I were to even make my opening lift, I had
to have the practice bench. I made the move for integration—not
out of morality but out of desperation, slipping onto the bench press
without even bothering to wait in line. Titanium approached me

after my warm-up sets. He had been *warming up* with 400 pounds. What he would do in the actual competition was beyond imagining.

"What you doin' here?" he asked, trailed by a few new friends in do-rags.

"What do you mean?" I said uneasily. A preppie among gang-bangers? A white among blacks?

"You ain't no powuhliftuh! You a bodybuilder, that's what I mean," he said, his friends nodding their heads behind him. They weren't angry, just confused.

It was true, I stuck out like a sore thumb. Unlike the powerlifters at this meet, I had legs, I didn't have a belly, and I had more veins running on the surface of my skin than most of them had underneath it. The veteran powerlifters in the group knew I wouldn't be as strong as I looked because I didn't train for strength. The beginners thought I'd be stronger than strong, because I *looked* it (and that's just what I'd been training for the last four years—that look, that appearance of strength). If I was a scream in search of a mouth, I'd chosen the wrong song.

When the hour struck, and the crowded court could hold no more, the judges with their colored paddles took their seats and the competition began. One by one, the lighter competitors filed out from the darkness at the sound of their names from the crackling PA system. As in bodybuilding shows, the lightweight classes went first, which left myself, Titanium, and a scattering of others the only remaining contestants at the warm-up bench. I planned on opening at 365, 40 pounds beneath my new Inzer Blast best, but a much higher weight than the maximum lifts in the lightest classes.

As a final preparation, I donned the Inzer Blast Shirt. Turbo and Titanium took turns stretching it onto my body. It was murder—more confining than a straitjacket, even worse than the first time with Macon and Lamar. But the pain vanished as soon as I heard my name on the PA system. It was adrenaline's turn. I dabbed my hands with chalk and emerged from the gloom with my arms strung out before me as if I were choking someone.

Mounting the dais, I spun around and lay down on the bench, arms extended upwards. Thirty inches above my face rested the bar laden with 365 solid pounds, a weight I paused without difficulty back at Shangri-La. But that was with an adequate warm-up, and not in front of three hundred people.

At my count of three, the two official spotters helped me lift the bending iron bar off the steel trestles, where I held it at arm's length. They let go. I was on my own now. At one with myself and iron. It didn't feel heavy. I let it slowly descend to my raised chest, then, keeping my bottom in continuous contact with the bench and my feet in unmoving contact with the ground, I paused the weight on my nipples. I waited for the clap for what seemed like three long agonizing seconds. I heard it at last and began the bar's ascent. Something was wrong. My progress slowed, and I realized I was in trouble. I heard a rising roar from the crowd. My face froze in terror, but I pushed with all my might, not stopping until I locked my arms out and threw the weight back onto the rack.

I rose from the bench unsteadily and eyed the judges to my right. The verdict was green. My opener was a success.

"My man!" Titanium said to me as I rejoined the others. In a flash, I understood. He had mistaken my interminable pause for arrogance, instead of what it really was—incompetence.

"What shows you done, man?" he asked.

"This is my first," I revealed, smiling. "How about you?"

"You know, here and there, FCI mostly," he said under his breath.

"FCI?" I was familiar with the governing bodies of powerlifting, the ADFPA (American Drug-Free Powerlifting Association), the USPF (United States Powerlifting Federation), the IPF (International Powerlifting Federation), and the WBPC (World Bench Press Congress), but I had never heard of FCI.

Titanium clued me in with a whisper. "Federal Correction Institution." He went on to admit with some pride that he held the all-time high for 242's at the Texas Federal Prison, Texarkana.

As politely as possible, I removed myself from Titanium to tell the record keeper of my second attempt, 385 pounds. All according to plan, first 365, then 385, and lastly, for glory, 405.

After only one round, the competition was gearing up in expected fashion. I had anticipated this much from *Powerlifting USA*. The best bench pressers were the competitors in the 181- and 198-

pound categories. Like my friend Hero, they combined large chests and short arms for startling results. In the state of California, the record holder for the bench in the 198-pound class, B. Ravenscroft, has lifted an astounding 581 pounds, while the record holder for the heavier weight class of 220 pounds has a personal best of 50 pounds less. I consoled myself with this fact as I watched men 50 pounds lighter than myself lifting one hundred pounds more than I could. If anything, my body was made for deadlifting. There, long arms and short legs are an advantage. Here, I was out of my element.

The PA system announced a short intermission, signaling the completion of the first round. I wandered to the door and stuck my head out, waving to my friends in attendance from the gym. Lamar, his Mohawk neatly trimmed by his father, was occupied by the carob bar in his hands and Cuddles in his lap. Moses nodded and smiled. Vinnie, standing on his chair, was pointing to the far corner of the room and shouting something at me.

I followed his finger and found the rest of the crowd congregating in the far corner of the gym. Standing behind a makeshift booth, I spotted a small, familiar figure. Where had I seen him before?

Why, it was Dr. Squat himself! Fred Hatfield, from the pages of *Powerlifting USA* and the Budweiser World Record Breakers—the first man in history to squat over a thousand pounds! In the magazines, looking stronger than an ox, he shook his fist to the sky in his STAND AND DELIVER T-shirt. I walked over and found him behind his booth, peddling his signature weight-lifting belts: The Thor, The Valhalla, and The Viking. I couldn't help notice, though, that in the flesh Dr. Squat looked less like a Teutonic warrior than a beleaguered and downtrodden Saxon villager. First, it was his weight. Seventy pounds lighter than in his championship days in Hawaii, he was drowning in his own clothes. Second was his hair. All that remained on his shiny noggin were a few scattered gray threads. Those dull and glazed eyes belonged on a dead fish. Judging by his appearance, the thousand-pound squat and the supplementing and force-feeding that had gone into it had nearly killed him.

But before I could so much as examine his American Power Belt, the second round began. I retreated to the warm-up room to practice a few light sets before my next attempt. I rubbed my palms and fingers with chalk to ensure a firm grip on the bar.

Vinnie joined me and helped Turbo and Titanium squeeze me into the Inzer Blast Shirt again. I tightened my wrist wraps. I heard my name on the PA system. It was all in the mind, I realized. I allowed no negative thoughts to enter my consciousness. Barreling through the doors into the raw sunlight, I felt an unshakable conviction. There was no stopping me. Not this time. I paused on the platform, the crowd murmured. I quickly spun around, arranged myself on the bench, and held my hands out at arm's length from my chest. Three hundred eighty-five pounds. I was ready.

I grabbed the steel bar in a flash and gripped it with everything I had, which sent chalk down to my face like sawdust in the sunlight. I counted to three, my spotters lifted the bar to my locked arms, and away I went. I gasped. It felt like a ton of bricks as it dove down to park on my chest. The clap, the clap, finally the clap. Up the bar flew. But now trouble. Two inches off my chest, it would not budge. I felt the crowd behind me, screaming.

"Like a human piston, Sam, like a human piston!" Macon shouted.

Right. A machine, clockwork, precision, unthinking, unfeeling. I caught my second wind and pushed.

"Lighter than a broomstick, Sam!" I heard Macon's shout again.

But it wasn't. It was heavier than a baby grand. Slowly, then with increasing speed, the bar headed back to my Adam's apple. The official spotters jerked it back onto the trestles.

In my disappointment, I kept my face averted from the crowd and made my way back to the other lifters in the warm-up room. They were full of commiseration. More than one contestant sought me out to inform me that I had nearly had it, that I was just an inch or two away from the initial lockout phase.

My technique, they said, was the problem. One of the 220's advised me: "Your first mistake: waiting on the fat man to clap. Don't wait, man, you got to anticipate the motherfucker."

A shorter lifter joined the argument: "That's right," he said, draping an arm around my shoulder. "You got to learn to cheat, man. Make the fat man work for *you!*"

The more I watched the other competitors, the more I realized that they were right. The best lifters, like Chip Taylor, brought the bar down to their chests and paused all right, but only for a second, not for two or three as I had done.

Immediately, I began my preparations for the third and final lift. I couldn't very well go on to 405 now—not after failing at 385. And as badly as I missed 385, I couldn't select a lower weight now, not according to powerlifting rules. That left 385 again.

I was no longer nervous, just infuriated. I had let everyone down. My self-disgust grew as I watched in the third and final round the 181's and 198's play with weights in the high 400's and, in one lifter's case, the low 500's. And I, all I could do was 365? Pathetic!

This was it. Once more, I applied liberal doses of chalk to my hands, my chest, my face, and bottom. Before I went on, Vinnie appeared in the warm-up room, doing his best to psych me up for the lift. Desperate times demanded desperate measures.

First, the "Heightened Arousal Mode." "Do the right thing, Vinnie!" I screamed, bracing myself for the worst. Vinnie tightened a black kid-leather lifting glove onto his hand, drew his fist back and delivered a blow so severe it sent me staggering.

Second, the Arnold Mental Visualization Principle, which I utilized on my wavering way to the bench press. I imagined myself in a "roid rage" crushing an infant's pacifier before his dewy eyes. Up on the platform, I was as ready as I could be. At the count of three, I snatched the bar from my spotters and let it drop down to my chest. It felt like nothing. I paused it professionally, and, a split second before hearing the clap, exploded upwards. Perfect. So close they couldn't call me on it.

My progress was steady. Seven inches, eight, nine. I was just entering the initial lockout phase, and I was still smiling. Suddenly, the bar stopped. Nothing worked, not my screams, not the wild buckling of my hips, not even Vinnie's encouraging roar ("EX-PLODE! EXPLODE!"). In the end, it was just too much. Again, the attendants grabbed the bar on its downward descent. The spectators gave me a polite round of applause, mostly spearheaded by the boys, I noticed.

In the trophy presentation that followed, all the lifters gathered in the first few rows with their relatives, friends, and fellow gym rats. The presentation, like the order of the lifting itself, was arranged by weight class. This meant Titanium and I watched together as the other competitors received their trophies first. The winner of the open division, by Schwartz Formula, was the 123-pound Chip Taylor who bench pressed nearly three times his body weight. Finally, the 242-pound class was announced.

Though there were two other competitors in my weight class, I was the first to be called to get my award. "And in third place . . ." Gus announced. Vinnie and the rest of the boys clapped madly, as I rose and did "the Walk" between the aisles to the podium. After all the three on, one offs, the supplementing, the food, the drugs, at last I had a trophy to tell me just who and what I was.

When I reached Gus, he covered the microphone with a massive paw, bent slightly in my direction, and whispered in my ear: "Look son, we had more competitors than we thought in your weight class. We thought you'd enter as a 275. So this is the best we can do. Sorry about that, Stan." He patted my rump sympathetically, and handed me a plaque on which were inscribed in gold plate the words:

Women 148 lbs
First Place

11.

THE BLITZ

---

*IT OFTEN OCCURRED TO HIM THAT IT WAS ALL
PROBABLY MEANINGLESS ANYWAY, A KIND OF
GAME. BUT IF IT TOOK A GAME TO KEEP HIM
ALIVE, SO BE IT.*

—HARRY CREWS

My disappointment at the Ninth Annual Rose City Bench-Press Extravaganza, my narrow escape from "bombing"—there was no time to consider any of this now. I had just six weeks until the Mr. San Gabriel Valley, and then, a week after that, the Mr. Golden Valley. Most bodybuilders give themselves 10 to 12 weeks of preparation for the contest countdown. With only half the time, I would have to work twice as hard.

Vinnie couldn't stress it enough when I met him and Nimrod, veterans both of many muscle wars, for a power conference at Shangri-La. "Big Man," he said, grabbing my arm and looking directly into my eyes, "it's time to end the larval stage and emerge a butterfly, a butterfly with big man muscles and a competition tan."

Vinnie told me not to panic if I didn't gain any more size before the contest. The goal, now, wasn't to get bigger: there was too little time for that. It was simply to *appear* to be bigger. And the only way to achieve this muscular *trompe l'oeil* was by improving the quality of my muscle and by losing fat, 15 to 20 pounds of it, in fact.

Vinnie had just the means to achieve this transformation. He waved a piece of paper above his head and slammed it down on the table before me. Carefully calibrated by himself and Nimrod, it was my dietary chart for 5½ of the next 7 weeks.

It read:

Menu	Amount	Calories	Protein	Fat	Carbohydrates	Sodium
Breakfast						
Eggs, poached	2	164	12.8	11.6	.8	272
Whole Wheat Bread	2 slices	122	5.2	1.6	24.0	266
Snack						
Apple	1 medium	85	.5	1.0	20.5	2
Lunch						
Tuna	6 ounces	254	56.0	1.6	000	82
Baked Potato	1 medium	142	4.0	.2	32.1	6
Dinner						
Chicken Breast	½ medium	160	26.0	5.1	000	64
Sweet Potato	1 medium	161	2.4	.6	37.1	14
Totals		1,088	106.9	21.7	114.5	696

All the joys of my five-thousand-calorie-a-day habit were gone. No more milk, not even nonfat milk. It was deemed nutritionally wasteful for competition. No more protein shakes. They were far too caloric. No more red meat. In fact, there would be practically no more anything, even tap water (whose sodium content was too high).

The aim of this diet was to keep my fat and sodium levels to a minimum, while juggling my carbohydrate to protein ratio. The juggling would start in the final 10 days before the contest. First, I would have to deplete my carbs and add slightly more protein. Then, 4 days before the contest, I would suddenly reverse the procedure, carbo-loading. It was a fine line. Not enough carbs, and I'd end up looking anemic. Too many, and I'd look bloated.

If I timed it right, on the day of the contest my skin would look as tight as a drum. Bodybuilders call it the "shrink-wrap" fit. According to Nimrod, it was the only way "to show your finer aesthetic qualities, your intercostals, the cross-striations on your quadriceps and triceps heads."

It was imperative that I start my diet immediately. The effect of elasticized parchment paper for skin can be obtained only gradually. As Vinnie said, "Too much weight lost too quickly leaves you with loose folds of skin on the posin' dais. It'll make you look like a Sharpei dog."

But Vinnie and Nimrod knew that my body weight probably wouldn't be a problem. Even after increasing my red meat intake for the strength contest, my fat content was abnormally low for a bodybuilder off-season. The mystery was what I would look like after this diet. Some bodybuilders lose their muscles along with their fat from forced weight loss. What with their fake tans and long, strandy ropes for muscles, they look like turbanned fakirs. Come contest time, would I have any muscles and muscle shape left?

One way to improve my muscle shape was to temporarily halt my steroid program. Vinnie instructed me to conclude my injectables, the testosterone and the Deca a full 10 days before the contest, since both drugs have a reputation for causing water retention. The orals, the Anavar, could be used up to 7 days before the contest.

But I didn't worry about going off—not yet, anyway (the psychological ramifications of that would come later). I worried about staying on for the next 7 weeks. What with my preparations for the strength contest, 16 straight weeks seemed an exceptionally long cycle to me, but not to Vinnie, who clued me in on the boys and girls of Venice.

"Shit, Big Man, some of those eighteen-wheelers don't go off for a full year. Compared to them, you're cleaner than a Safeway chicken. . . . "

So, while Tara fretted about her vocational future behind Shangri-La's counter ("I mean, like, it's between industrial psychology, you know how I am with people, or like, equestrian therapy . . . I mean, I'm really excellent with kids, too"), I set about meeting my own destiny.

From seven to nine every morning, and again from five to seven every evening, I fell back into my by now old habit of three on, one off training, with one major exception. It was now seven on, none off, a perpetual recycling. I couldn't afford the luxury of rest days. The first morning, it was chest and shoulders, that night, biceps and triceps, the next morning, quads, the next night, calves and hamstrings, the next morning, back and traps, that night shoulders and forearms, ad infinitum. Abs every day. Five hundred reps, broken down into ten sets of 50, took an extra 30 minutes. After the excursion into powerlifting training, it was a relief to return to my old schedule.

In order to shed my veneer of fat and show raw muscle, I blasted through my sets with higher repetitions, at least 15 to 20, which necessitated lower weight. Instead of fifteen sets per body part, the powerlifting norm, I increased it to twenty-five or thirty and concentrated on working the muscle rather than just heaving heavy poundages. The exercises were similar, but the approach was radically different.

Back at my desk in New York, I'd seen a black-and-white photograph of the enormous Arnold doing lateral shoulder raises with a 15-pound weight. I had thought it incredible at the time—such a big man, such a little weight. Now I knew, thanks to Vinnie and Nimrod, that come contest time, these smaller weights were just the thing to slice off fat and reveal underlying muscle size and shape. Contest preparation involves endurance, not strength.

"Train Big, Eat Big, Sleep Big" became "Train Longer and Lighter, Eat Less and Wisely, and Sleep Whenever Possible." After just 2 weeks of this intensified program, I was training so hard and eating so little that I no longer had energy for anything. Personal training had to go. I informed Moët and Mr. and Mrs. Slatkin and all my other clients that I would be unavailable for the duration. It worked out well for Moët—she was going in for surgery for a quick boob and bottom touch-up and would be incapacitated for the next month as a result anyway. Bamm Bamm temped for me with the others.

Throughout my training sessions, I clung to my visualization principles. Vinnie had won the Golden Valley three years earlier, and on his wall at home hung the fruits of that labor. It was a glorious silver saber (the cusped hilt trimmed in red velvet), awarded to the overall winner of the show. A bronze plaque was affixed to the radiant scabbard, the inscription commemorating Vinnie as builder and man.

I also clung to my clichés. "Formula for success, a straight line, a goal," was my muscle mantra, penned by that gym favorite, Friedrich Nietzsche. And underneath those great blown-up images of

Raoul that hung from the rafters, I recited that mantra until it was an unintelligible whisper as I set about reinventing myself. I will become the person I want to be, I vowed. I will elongate my bicep with preacher curls, I will add to the outside sweep of my quads with the aid of the hack squat machine and a close-grip stance. I will enlarge my neck with the neck harness. I will become a body-builder.

But while I kept visualizing the saber and eyeing Raoul up above, I couldn't help but see myself in the many mirrors of Shangri-La. I examined my frame while I was changing, while I was pumping out reps, while I was sipping from my bottle of distilled water. The mirror was vital now, according to Vinnie, to be used for an instantaneous progress report.

To be used, in fact, as much as the Medco was to be avoided. Watching the scale register my weight loss could stop me from dieting. To weigh myself would be counterproductive, would confuse mass with class, Vinnie said. My weight was irrelevant. All that mattered was the mirror; it would tell me everything I needed to know. But as I trained in quest of the silver saber, the mirror told me more than I wanted to know.

"Bodybuilding. It's not just about size, it's about symmetry," was a line as common in the gym as in the magazines. "The Apollonian Ideal," this symmetry was called, after classical Greek sculpture. The neck, the calves, the arms should all be the same size. Ideally, for a man my height, each should measure 20 inches. To be in proper proportion, my chest should measure 60 inches, my waist 32, and my thighs 30 (half my chest).

As the San Gabriel Valley approached, the mirror attested that I was decidedly asymmetrical. My calves were 17 inches, my arms 18, my neck 19. My chest at 52 inches was not twice my thighs (at 28 inches each). My waist was 34, not 32. As a result, I found myself in the gym every day for 5 hours feverishly playing catch-up, trying to bring up my lagging body parts. The more I worked, the more I panicked when one body part started to outdistance another.

Vinnie did his best to calm me down. The judges do not tape-measure physique competitors, he reminded me, they simply examine them from a distance of 20 feet. A bodybuilder with 18-inch arms can make them look better than a rival with 20 inches, if he knows how to show them to the judges and audience. And what if I *was* a long way off from the ideal? I wasn't, after all, entering a professional contest, merely the San Gabriel Valley and the Golden Valley a week later. But all that was little consolation. As I saw it, if I wasn't symmetrical, I wasn't really a bodybuilder, and if I wasn't a bodybuilder, then what exactly was I?

Judging by the mirror, I was a bodybuilder from the 1950s. I was light-years beyond Sandow at the turn of the century. I was even better than the first great builders, John Grimek and Clancy Ross from the 1940s. But by the fifties, bodybuilding had caught up with me. Steve Reeves had me on symmetry and aesthetics, Bill Pearl on size. I was no match for Schwarzenegger and the other bodybuilding greats of the sixties, Sergio Oliva and Larry Scott, much less the giants, like Lee Haney, who had evolved since then.

No, to be considered one of the best bodies in the world, I would have to go back thirty years. Back then, 18-inch arms like mine were halfway between Charles Atlas and Arnold. But it was 1988, not 1958, and now I would be hard-pressed to win even a local contest like Mr. San Gabriel Valley.

Still, if I didn't win, it wouldn't be for lack of effort. I didn't play catch-up only in the gym, I did it even in my own bedroom. Every other night, I woke up, reached under my bed, and pulled out a 25-pound dumbbell. Lying as still as possible, I did ten sets of lateral raises for each shoulder (in the hope that the bigger my deltoids grew the smaller my waist would look). After 15 sweaty minutes, I had just enough energy to drop the weight and, exhausted, fall asleep.

I was gripped by a kind of muscle madness, both in the gym and out. On the sidewalks outside Shangri-La, I couldn't see my shadow without gagging. It looked so elongated as it stretched out before me. Did I really look like that? Like ET with a gym bag? And the suspicions raised by my shadow were confirmed by my clothes. As the weeks before the contest passed and I continued to shrink, my clothes took on increasingly Brobdingnagian proportions. I understood at last those bodybuilders who announced their miraculous "muscle gains" as they weighed themselves fully clothed in hooded sweatshirts, lifting belts, and construction boots.

Often, I checked in the mirror to make sure I was still all there, that the "real" me, the puffery and muscles, was still me. The more I trained to keep that "real" me, that Michelin Man me, the more I realized the cruel nature of bodybuilding. At any given moment, some of your muscles are growing, yes. But the obverse is also true: At any given moment, some of your muscles are atrophying. According to sports physiologists, a muscle left dormant for 72 hours is a muscle that, unused, unneeded, begins to vanish.

In order to obtain "maximum growth," as they say in the gym, I had to store in my mind a perpetual mental timetable of just what muscle I'd worked when, in order to keep from drying up and blowing away. In effect, I was caught up in a solipsistic game of tag with my own muscles.

But this catch-up game wasn't just about my lagging body parts. It was also about my age.

"You like the music this loud?" I'd said to Vinnie that first day I trained with him two years earlier. I'd had to shout to be heard above the din of his Walkman.

"Sam," he responded, shouting himself, "if it's too loud, you're too old."

It all seemed easy enough for Arnold, who had started lifting at fifteen. But I had started at twenty-six, and no matter how often I brought up Chuck Sipes, Ed Corney, and others who had made it late, I was concerned enough about my age to lie about it constantly. No great bodybuilder had ever started as late as I had. My age was one part of me I couldn't control, couldn't reinvent. What if all this was for nought? Not just these contests, but beyond. The logical sequence dictated that after Mr. Golden Valley, I would progress to Mr. Los Angeles; from Mr. LA, I'd move on to Mr. California, then to the Nationals, and finally to the Pros.

The time I didn't spend training or worrying about my shadow, my shoulders, my diminution, or my age, I worried about the actual competition.

According to Vinnie, a bodybuilding show consisted of: the morning Prejudging, which included Round One—the preliminary line-up; Round Two—mandatory or compulsory poses; and Round Three—free posing (60 seconds, without music), and, then, "The Evening Show"; the line-up once more; the posing routine (90 seconds to music); the pose-down; and, for the winners of each particular weight class, the pose-down for the overall title.

Vinnie didn't bother me with the details concerning each element of the show. Instead, he wholeheartedly helped me with my posing, which I practiced every afternoon before the critical eyes of all three of my roommates.

First, there were the mandatories to learn, those eight standards I'd aped from the magazines long ago in front of the lavatory's mirror at work. The judges would call for these poses for comparison shots. We took them one at a time, with Vinnie and Nimrod twisting and plying my limbs into the appropriate flexed postures. I learned how to contort my body into (1) the front-lat spread; (2) the side chest; (3) the side triceps; (4) the front double-biceps; (5) the back double-biceps; (6) the back-lat spread; (7) the leg extended, hands behind head, abdominal pose; and (8) the most muscular.

Second, there was the posing routine itself, in which these moves and more are incorporated into 90 seconds. Ninety seconds during which the builder makes one clockwise or counterclockwise full circle to music, stopping at certain points along the way to display his physique from the front, the side, the back, the other side, and the front again.

For my music, I chose 90 seconds of "Theme from Shaft" by Isaac Hayes. It had everything I wanted: a slow, haunting beginning rising to a loud, energetic beat, finally triggering a violent, string crescendo for my crabs.

Professional bodybuilders take as long as three minutes to show their physiques. With the added time, their routines are more intricate than one counterclockwise turn. But I didn't have three minutes. I had half that, and I planned on fitting just ten major poses within that time; two each at six o'clock, three o'clock, twelve o'clock, nine o'clock, and six o'clock again.

To begin, I chose (1) "Giant in Respose." Down on one knee, I cast my head at my feet, and pushed my left bicep against my raised other knee to make my arm appear fuller.

Then, as the music began, I rose. "Like the fuckin' orchid, ya bloom!" this never failed to evoke from Vinnie.

Standing in the six o'clock position, I expanded into (2) the front-lat spread. I kept my heels together, bent my knees slightly, and held my hands slightly above my obliques.

One-quarter turn to my left, and I stood at three o'clock. Looking back over my right shoulder, I hit (3) the side chest, which displayed my tightened upper torso.

Still at three o'clock, I pushed my arms out away from my body and kept them parallel to one another, at right angles to the rest of my torso. This was (4) the arms extended pose. When Arnold did it, his biceps looked like loaves of bread. Mine looked like two sausage links.

One-quarter turn again to my left and I stood at twelve o'clock, with my back to the stage. The perfect position to raise my arms and display my shoulders, arms, and trapezius muscles in (5) the back double-biceps. Judges can detect the shape of a builder by the quality of his "Christmas tree," the spinal erectors, from this position.

Still at twelve o'clock, I flexed into (6) the back-lat spread. Instead of keeping my arms upraised and flexed, I held my hands at my hips, and stretched the wings of my latissimus dorsi, while simultaneously tightening my calf muscles.

One more quarter turn to my left and I stood at nine o'clock. Since my right bicep had a higher peak and overall better size than my left, I shot two poses from this angle: (7) the one arm extended bicep pose and (8) "Hair." The first involved keeping my left arm close to my body to make it look fuller. With a slight twist to the left to expose my upper chest, I raised my slightly crooked right arm almost to shoulder level, and, keeping it away from my body, flexed it. A singular loaf of bread, in theory.

Then, still standing at nine o'clock, I moved my left arm upward, passed it over my hair, while simultaneously smiling and flexing my now fully raised right bicep. The pose called "Hair" necessitates a gleaming smile and an addiction to the life and gestures of body-builder Tom Platz.

One last turn, and I was back at six o'clock, completing the counterclockwise circle and facing the audience.

With but 15 seconds left, there was just time for (9) the legs extended, hands overhead, ab shot ("Garbo") and (10) the most muscular variation ("Crabs"). "Garbo" I performed by holding my head in my hands in Steichen fashion, and flexing my abdominal muscles and thighs. The "Crabs" were the perfect finale, bringing all my blood to the surface in a hideous display of beef bordering on spontaneous combustion.

Diagrammed, the whole routine looked like this:

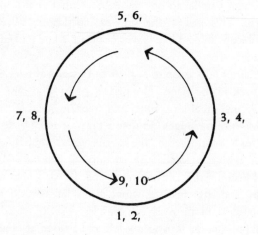

In the free-posing round, there are two vital maneuvers to consider: first, the actual poses, and second, the transitional moves into and out of those poses. You need to twist on your feet without stumbling or windmilling your arms for balance. Up on the high wire, the trapeze artist frantically waves his arms to generate a feeling of danger. But on the dias, the goal is to generate safety, security. The bodybuilder projects a feeling of utter self-control. The winner in the free-posing round is not simply the man with the best body, but the builder most adept at selling the fantasy. And since these are muscle shows, it is power and brute force, along with grace and style, that rock the crowd.

Aside from projecting pure emotive force, I had to learn tricks; what to accentuate, what to hide. Up on stage, every bodybuilder is an illusionist, always armed with artifice to cast his spell. By never locking the legs, the quads look fuller and larger. By keeping the feet at an angle with heels joined, the calves look bigger. I had to keep my bent legs together to make them appear thicker from the side.

Just as important as the size and quality of my muscles was the ability to display them. I needed to show my physique to *all* the seated judges, not just those stage center, but those seated to the far left or right as well. So every pose necessitated a hip swivel. Too many bodybuilders rush through their posing, which is infuriating for the audience. To maintain a slow rhythm, Vinnie advised me to count out loud. "One, two, swivel, three, four, swivel, five, shift, pose, smile." "One, two, swivel, three, four, swivel, five, shift, pose, smile." Again and again and again.

Memorizing the whole routine took days. Making the whole thing look joyful and spontaneous, instead of the mapped-out, scripted, well-rehearsed essay it is, took weeks. From my entrance on stage to my exit, it was *all* rehearsed. My entrance was stolen from Arnold's 1975 Olympia in Pretoria, South Africa. On his walk to the dais, he flicked an imaginary bead of sweat from his massive upper pecs to draw the attention of the judges to the area. My concluding bow was stolen from Tom Platz's appearance at the 1980 Olympia in Sydney, Australia.

My routine was dramatic, all right, but not too dramatic. The goal is to play by the audience's accepted rules, and then to shock them within the form, not venturing outside it. Michelangelo's *David* and the Farnese *Hercules* are one thing, but, as professional bodybuilder Bob Paris learned, *The Dying Gaul* is quite another. From the Capitoline Museum in Rome to Columbus, Ohio, Paris concluded his posing program with *The Dying Gaul* at the 1989 Arnold Classic. It was met with an uncomfortable silence and angry suspicion, the latter confirmed months later when he revealed his marriage to his "husband," male model Rod Jackson, and the joy they shared in their "children," two dogs and a Macaw named Barney.

Ten days before the contest, I looked less like a bodybuilder than a football player. I was still carrying too much water, so Vinnie shut down my carbohydrates, not completely, but on a 55 percent protein, 35 percent carbs, 10 percent fat split. Without carbs, I had no energy left to wade through my workouts, so the boys took turns training with me. Some sessions, it was Lamar (with Macon pressing us on), others Vinnie, still others Nimrod or G-spot.

As the event grew closer, my most pressing waking consideration, aside from training, became my tan and tracking down the best methods to achieve it. The definition I had sculpted into my body in the previous weeks would be undetected without the glow of a healthy tan. I needed the sun to keep my fish belly white body from looking flat and fat under the harsh lights of the stage. But the sun wouldn't be enough. As Nimrod accurately foretold, my WASP genes would also necessitate daily tanning sessions from Shangri-La's sun bed.

Thus, I spent 30 minutes before my workout each morning sequestered in the cocoon of the tanning bed. There I sat in a cradle of brilliant light, my naked hulking body stretched out before me, exposed to the humming rays I rented to penetrate my skin. But despite daily sessions, the first week passed without any result whatsoever. I increased the radiation dosage from a half hour to an hour per session. Still no result. Just as I feared, the problem was not with the machine, but with my own stubborn skin.

In desperation, in the final days before the contest, I purchased a trunk load of tanning products from a retail bodybuilding outlet in West Covina called The Health Factory. Pro-Tan Instant Competition Color. Dye-O-Derm with special sponge-applicator tip. Part alcohol, part brown dye, I was fine so long as I avoided open fires or furniture. I could touch nothing without befouling it with my competition color. The chairs, the walls, the La-Z-Boy, the knobs on the television set, the toilet seat, the dishes—I made my mark on them all.

And though the products, as they warned, completely clogged my skin, adding to the collection of carbuncles and whiteheads I acquired through my supplementation program, the brown coatings finally stuck (provided I didn't shower or wear a full suit of clothing).

Three days before the show, Vinnie finally flushed my body with carbohydrates. After so many weeks on 1,000 calories a day, it was a relief to carbo-load for my last four days. I substituted oatmeal and raisins for my two eggs and a slice of bread for breakfast, and was allowed a side of spaghetti for a midafternoon snack.

As the training and dieting and varnishing took effect, the result, two days out before the contest, was indisputable. The mirror did not lie. I had effected a most extraordinary mutation. The man staring back at me was, unquestionably, a bodybuilder. With the reduction of my waistline and the tightening of my abdominal muscles, my chest looked twice its normal size. Veins covered my thighs and chest like cobwebs. Thanks to my diet, my skin was thinner than airmail paper. And with my varnish, I was browner than a buried pharaoh. I've done it, I thought to myself. I've actually done it. I had at last achieved the metamorphosis. What my father called "an atavistic nightmare," what Clive James called "a condom filled with walnuts," what my mother called "a cautionary conceit," I had become. A bodybuilder at last.

Those bronzed, muscle-bound figures in the glossy magazine pages had always seemed to me creatures from another world, in some way not quite human. And God only knew, how many hours, how many days, how many years I had spent trying to join their ranks.

Then why did I feel so awful? Thanks to the rigors of my training, my hands were more ragged, callused and cut than any longshoreman's. Thanks to the drugs and my diet, I couldn't run 20 yards without pulling up and gasping for air. My ass cheeks ached from innumerable steroid injections, my stomach whined for sustenance, my whole body throbbed from gym activities and enforced weight-loss. Thanks to the competition tan, my skin was breaking out everywhere. Vinnie and Nimrod explained that all this was perfectly normal.

"What, do you think this has anything to do with health?" Nimrod asked, shaking in mirth at the idea.

"Big Man, this is about *looking* good, not feeling good," Vinnie added soberly.

But it wasn't simply my shortness of breath that bothered me, or my accelerated heart rate, dizziness, or bruised hands. No, I suffered from a more severe affliction, and well I knew it. I'd become a bodybuilder to be comfortable with a self I'd invented. I had counted on the security, the simplicity of the mask, the armor. But once I'd manufactured all the muscles and the puffery, I felt trapped inside this colossal frame. Everywhere I went, I heard myself breathe. I didn't need to see passersby doing double takes to be aware of my own movements, to watch myself—this huge, ungainly creature, suffocated by a world of his own making. In the end, "the Walk" I did, the being I had become, felt stifling, limiting, claustrophobic, far from liberating, as it had once been on the corner of Fifty-third and Second back in New York.

But no one in Shangri-La detected a thing. To them, with my muscles and my new competition color, I was a rank and file body-builder. Opinion was divided on the expected outcome of the contest. Some gym rats, hearing the quantity of drugs I had consumed in my efforts, labeled me "The Experiment," in homage to a college football player whose steroid exploits had just then made the pages of *Sports Illustrated*. They were convinced that no one could stop me from winning both my weight class and the overall trophy. They saw my victory as a product of science.

Others were convinced that by entering the open class, I had invited disaster: that only a fool would compete in an unlimited class in his first venture on the stage. Hadn't I, after all, come close to "bombing" at the strength exhibition?

But I was deaf to everything. To keep from feeling bad, I kept myself from feeling anything at all. Nothing penetrated my muscular armor. I had descended completely into a world of my own, a world based on sets and reps, anabolic steroids and vitamin supplementation, coats of Pro-Tan and Dye-O-Derm, compulsory and optional poses, and protein and carb and sodium and fat ratios.

12.

THE SAN GABRIEL VALLEY

THE MUSCLE-FLEXING IS OFTEN THERE, ALL RIGHT, AND IT IS REAL, BUT IT IS NOT, AS SO MANY ASSUME, BORN OF A DESIRE TO BE TOUGH.

—*JAMES M. CAIN*

By the time I heard Vinnie's knock, I had already been up and posing for an hour. I counted on last-minute isometric squeezing and flexing to increase my vascularity and muscle separation for prejudging.

"You ready, Big Man?"

I checked my Gold's Gym bag. Original Muscle-Up Professional Posing Oil? Check. Muscle Sheen? Check. Pro-Tan Instant Competition Color? Check. Sponge applicator tips? Check. Matte black competition briefs? Check. Mousse? Check. Sony Walkman? Check. A tape of my posing music? Check. A duplicate tape? Check.

"Your food?"

A Spartan mix of sodium-free rice cakes? Check. A half a cup of raisins? Check. A bottle of distilled water? Check. An anemic-looking boiled chicken breast? Check. A Tupperware cup of tasteless oatmeal? Check.

I looked up from my bag at Vinnie. "There will be no judges," I said. Vinnie beamed.

"Oh yes!" he screamed on the way to the car, "ring the alarm bell, ring it loud!"

Once inside the Luv, he stomped on the accelerator, before I could so much as fasten my do-rag over my moussed flattop. On that wild ride to the auditorium in El Monte we slowed down only once—for an elementary school child who had lost his jacks on the intersection in front of us. Vinnie veered toward the lad and, as I screamed, missed him by inches. He broke into an ear-splitting grin. The day was coming up roses for him already. I only hoped it would prove as wonderful for me.

But the fact was I didn't feel very wonderful. Though I hadn't had a shot in a week, my bottom still ached from my steroid injections. Of late, the needle felt like it was grinding against the bone. I hadn't taken a bath or a shower in a week in order to preserve my competition color. And my haircut, yes, there was my haircut. At the last moment, I had requested as close a crop as possible in the belief that the smaller my head looked, the bigger my body would appear.

But the barber had botched the job, leaving my flattop more tilted than a skateboard ramp, and now I wondered just how the judges would react when I made my entrance. As every bodybuilder in Shangri-La had told me, judges were unpredictable. The one thing I knew was that they would be seated behind a long table located in the space before the front row in the auditorium. They would look for muscle size, muscle definition, pleasing bone structure, symmetry, and charisma. Not necessarily in that order—in fact, in no order at all. Bodybuilding judging, like the sport itself, is still in its infancy.

When we parked outside the junior high school auditorium, I caught my first sight of my competitors. Most of them were clad in the same attire as my own: oversized terry-cloth tops and Gold's Gym sweats. Inside, the theater was utterly empty. It is only iron addicts of the most extreme kind who attend the morning prejudging. Depending on the number of contestants, these preliminaries can extend for as long as six or seven hours.

Beyond the heads of my entourage, I spotted a lone, tanned figure smiling to himself. A man in his sixties, he was seated in the front row, in the middle of the judges' panel. He looked as fit and competition-colored as he had thirty-five years earlier when he won his first Mr. America title, as he looked, in fact, in Leonard's imitation wood frame. It was Bill Pearl, whom no less a source than *The Encyclopedia* lists as "one of the greatest bodybuilders of all time."

Aside from the America, he had won the Mr. Universe title four times (spanning three different decades). If Arnold is bodybuilding's favorite son, Bill Pearl is its patron saint.

At the sound of the loudspeaker announcing the beginning of registration, I joined the line with my muscular kindred backstage. Most were teenage boys of every shape and size. My flattop haircut was the style of choice, in homage to Schwarzenegger and his latest cinematic epic, *Commando*. Others sported "rat tails" hanging down the back of the neck. One misguided fellow had instructed his barber to shave what looked like lightning bolts onto the hair covering each temple. Combined with the effect of his physique, which was both sagging and turgid, his haircut brought to mind shock therapy, rather than Mount Olympus.

I stood a head taller than all of them, bronzed, the very picture of health. The audience wouldn't know that my breathing was shallow, my heart rate abnormally high. The judges wouldn't hear my panting and puffing. I hoped Nimrod was right, and that the eruptions of my riotous complexion would be invisible under the glare of the stage lights. If he was wrong, I was sunk.

Immediately after registration, we filed off to a backstage room for the weigh-in. I stared over at the Medco in the corner. I hadn't weighed myself in six weeks. Each competitor took his turn on it according to weight class and division. First the teenagers, then the novices, then the open men, which meant, at last, the heavyweights.

As competitor after competitor stripped and mounted the scale, it was obvious that builders like to train the *front* of their bodies—the parts they face in the mirror. I saw good chests, quadriceps, and arms, but bad backs, hamstrings and calves—and I was no exception.

At the call for heavyweights, I peeled off everything but my competition briefs and valiantly strode to the Medco. There were whispers when Spanky, the meet organizer, announced my weight: 232 pounds! Twenty pounds more than anyone else in the show! I felt, on substance alone, I'd already won. I put my sweats back on while the others took to the scale. There were just three entrants in my weight class, and unlike the bench-press extravaganza, now I felt cheated. Now I wanted the competition.

The two other heavyweights were both black, but there the similarity ended. One was short and fat, the other tall and thin. Bursting with confidence, I walked out of the room with my lats spread as wide as I could flex them. I made sure that the other competitors noticed how difficult it was for me to squeeze through the door frame.

Peeking from behind the stage's red curtain, I saw Vinnie, seated with Macon, Lamar, Nimrod, and G-spot. I jauntily gave the thumbs-up sign to Nimrod, who elbowed Vinnie, who returned my gesture with an imploring one of his own. They needed to speak to me, it was obvious. What could it be? Something I'd taken? A toxic combination of steroids?

No, they were worried about the tall black contestant, the heavy-weight I had dismissed on the scale as not being in my league. According to Nimrod, who had seen him warming up, he was in many respects my superior and stood a good chance of winning the whole show.

"Look, Big Man," Vinnie explained breathlessly, his face inches from mine, "you got 'em on legs, but not on back and abs, so don't get in no comparison shots on abs, he's shredded."

"And remember," Vinnie added, "you want your place in the bodybuildin' pantheon? Well then, by golly, think smart and flex your legs next to his in the comparison rounds!"

Nimrod nodded his head. "And the most-musculars, Vinnie, don't forget the most-musculars."

"Right, right!" Vinnie cried. The teens were almost on stage. As the theater lights dimmed and Nimrod beat a hasty retreat to his seat, Vinnie dabbed a bit of Dye-O-Derm on my upper pecs and clapped me on the back.

"Remember, Sam, you don't get a second chance to make a good first impression!"

With this in mind, I dashed off to the official pump-up room. It was actually an enormous, backstage men's room, in which a crate of dumbbells and barbells had been placed in preparation for our exhibition. We had to put our dumbbells down on the white tiles carefully, so they wouldn't roll down the sloping floor into the trough of the urinal by the far wall.

Here, between the sink and the stalls, I stripped off the last of my layers and coated my body with Original Muscle-Up Professional Posing Oil. This would keep my muscles from looking flat under the glare of the lights. I pinned my number 9 to my black posing trunks. From a distance, it looked like a price tag. I dabbed the mousse I retrieved from my Gold's Gym bag onto my hair. There were forty bodybuilders in the bathroom, about ten more than it could comfortably accommodate.

I tried to ignore the grunting and groaning around me and grabbed the first weight that became available. Blocking everyone else out, I concentrated on performing repetition after repetition for my arms and shoulders, chest and calves. Everything but the thighs and the hamstrings, muscles which lose their definition when pumped.

Every ten minutes, a group of competitors left for the stage, until finally the vast room housed only the male open heavyweight competitors. I warmed up furiously now, my skin ready to burst from the force of the muscles and veins seething just beneath the skin. I flexed my best shots in front of one of the available mirrors, spying on my competitors out of the corner of my eye. This time, my eyes did not deceive me. The shorter of the two black men was history. He was big all right, but bloated. Everything was swollen, not just his muscles, but his cheeks, his forehead, his knuckles. Whether it was testosterone or Twinkies, the sodium in his body left him looking like a float in the Macy's Thanksgiving Day Parade.

But Nimrod and Vinnie were right. The taller builder flexing beside me, number 10, was good, there was no doubt about it. No dirigible, he. His abs were perfect, a regular washboard. His waist was half the size of mine, but my shoulder width was twice his. I was bigger everywhere, including some of the wrong places, like my obliques and hips. I had him on muscles; he had me on shape.

I looked down at one of the brown-stained index cards in my hand. Vinnie had given me a set, "for motivation of the warrior," he'd said. "RADIATE CONFIDENCE!" it read. I jutted my lats out a little further and practiced what I hoped would be taken for a spontaneous smile. Another index card: "THEY'VE COME TO BEAT YOU. YOU OWN THE CROWN."

"Open Heavyweights, you're on," a voice cried down the hall. Not a minute too soon. I made a last-minute check that my number was pinned to my trunks, and followed the others out the door. Dripping with oil and sweat, the three of us trailed the stage manager in silence to the curtain's edge. We waited for the signal from the assistant across the stage, and at the lowering of his arm, we filed out in numerical order.

Suddenly I remembered my last appearance on a stage. The blinding glare of the spotlights was the same, as was the air of expectation from the whispering crowd. Then, I wore a cardboard crown and pulled a stuffed camel on wheels. It was a Nativity scene, and I was in the second grade. Now, twenty years later, I stood before audience and judges in briefs, a number, and a tan.

As the three of us did "the Walk" toward stage center, I could just make out Bill Pearl's outline beyond the glare of the lights. At his direction, we stood in the line-up one arm's length from each other. In this round the judges would be checking for symmetry (that "Apollonian Ideal"), size, and "flow," the look the best builders have, of each body part flowing into the next, the look it takes years to develop, the look that none of us had.

I couldn't see Vinnie, but I heard him. "Spread 'em, Big Man!" he screamed from out there in the darkness. I cursed myself, still smiling pleasantly, and flexed everything I had, though we hadn't yet begun the mandatories. We were still "standing relaxed," but only a neophyte to the bodybuilding world would mistake the position for the dictionary definition.

"Standing relaxed" is, in fact, a bald-faced lie. It should be called "continuous tension," since it necessitates simultaneously squeezing the calves, the quads, the abs, the chest, the shoulders, the arms, and the lats, while maintaining the coolest of smiles. The weeks before the contest had seen my whole body convulse in reaction to the posture, but the practice had paid off. I could hold the position for 15 minutes, if necessary. I would not lose this round.

"Gentlemen, a quarter turn to your left, please," Mr. Pearl requested after just 3 minutes.

We "stood relaxed" from the side, a quarter turn more, with our backs to the audience, a quarter turn more, from the other side, a quarter turn more, again the front.

Finally, Mr. Pearl led us through the first of the eight mandatory poses. After all the afternoons spent in practice with Vinnie and Nimrod and Bamm Bamm, I couldn't have been better prepared for these. I remembered to keep my heels together, my knees slightly bent, and my thighs flared outwards for the front-lat spread. For the side-chest I turned my side to the audience, extended my arms outward, joined my hands, then brought them toward my chest with a resounding squeeze of my whole upper torso. Arnold had recommended this method of getting into the mandatory side-chest position in *The Encyclopedia*. A judge might call you on it, he said, but they'll love the drama. No one called me on it—the crowd was whooping and hollering.

One by one, the rest of the eight mandatories flew by. With only three of us on stage, the judges had no need to arrange us for tandem comparison as they noted the difference in our muscle separation, definition, and shape. At Mr. Pearl's order, two of us filed off to leave the stage to number 8, the shortest of all of us, for the silent, "free-posing" round.

Number 8 tried, but his 60-second round was received with dead calm by the audience. He left the stage visibly shaken by the experience. He told number 10 that he felt as if he'd just attended his own funeral.

I took the stage next and concentrated on looking both graceful and powerful, the latter easier to accomplish with my frame. For the "free-posing" round, I simply abbreviated the 90-second routine I planned to use that night, discarding poses that drew attention to my weak abs, inserting poses that highlighted my chest, shoulders, and quadriceps.

It couldn't have gone better. The applause started the moment I emerged from stage right with a confident grin, and didn't stop until the audience saw my heel disappear behind the curtain. By the time I reached the wings, I was glowing inside and out. But my whole body deflated when number 10 took the stage. With his smaller frame, he moved much more gracefully than I did; his confident air made it clear that, like me, he thought himself the winner. At the conclusion of his posing, for which he, too, received strong applause, the morning show ended. The audience left hastily to fit in a work-out and a meal before the real fun began.

Though most contests are actually decided in the morning, when the judges take the time needed to dissect minutely, then rank every competitor, the night show is the rowdy concession to the paying audience. Decorum is thrown out the window, and bodybuilders, heeding the pleas of the audience to "show us what you got!" are only too delighted to comply. After four years of labor, the ten minutes I stood on stage were it for the morning show. If I won my weight class that night, plus the overall trophy in the pose-down with the other weight-class winners that followed, I would be on stage for a maximum of 15 minutes more.

Back in the car, Vinnie knew that it was between me and number 10 for the heavyweight title. He was tall, black, and cut. I was taller, white, and more muscular—but also fatter. It depended on what the judges wanted that day, Vinnie said, cuts or size, the classic bodybuilding debate. Ideally, the perfect specimen of a body-builder should present the audience with both, but even on the Mr. Olympia stage, it is rare to find the ideal. From time immemorial, physique fans have argued on the absurdity of the contest itself. How, they ask, can you judge between a lily and a rose, between size and cuts, between competitors number 9 and number 10?

At Shangri-La that afternoon, the same argument raged around me as I bit my teeth into a quarter pound serving of orange roughy and drank two glasses of distilled water. At our power conference table by the juice bar, Macon prepared me for the possibility of defeat. He put an arm around Lamar, who had an arm around Cuddles.

With a troubled look, Macon sighed. "You know, Sam, you're like a second son to me, but, dagnabit, you never know which direction they'll go in. Why, back at Mr. Inland Empire last year, even Troy took second, remember Lamar? And to a pencil-neck!"

Lamar shook his head in disgust at the memory. I kept mum. I, too, knew it would be close that night.

"See, Sam," Macon explained, "it's not like you're not the biggest thing out there. Fact is, you are. Nimrod? Vinnie?" Vigorous nods from both. "It's just that you never can tell with the judges, I mean, examine history."

"Lamar?" Macon sat back and swallowed a Chewable.

Lamar, on cue, pressed forward from his seat. His enormous shape dwarfed Cuddles in his lap.

"Right, Dad," he intoned grimly. "Nineteen sixty-eight. Miami Beach Auditorium. Arnold came to America and lost the Universe—to Frank Zane, a man 70 pounds lighter, a human swizzle stick."

While Macon and Lamar shook their heads sadly at the injustice of it all, Nimrod and Vinnie were lost in thoughts of iron precedence.

Suddenly, Macon's face lit up. "Now, I'll tell you one thing Sam," he said, "that Bill Pearl is a real size queen, sure as I'm standing here today. He's an *American* builder, by golly, and I know as a fact you can count on his vote."

Everyone had advice for me that afternoon. I needed to concentrate on showing the muscle disparity between myself and number 10, and then to surprise the judges with some quality. I had good intercostals, considering my body weight, so Macon urged me to flex these when number 10 tried to hit his back shots.

Nimrod advised me to keep my head. "*Wemember*, man," Bamm Bamm chimed in, "no *diwect* back *compawison* shots. Keep to your *stwengths*, the arms and the *wegs*, then *wet* God sort out the fuckin' wounded."

"Jesus fuckin' Christ!" Vinnie screamed suddenly, rising from his seat. He could take no more. "What on earth is happening here? The time has come to get rid of pasty faces! Sam, at the warm-up tonight, you just show them who's who, OK? Buddy, you want to pulverize that number 10 tonight? Then you grab 'im, Sam, and you shake 'im by his balls!"

When we arrived back at the theater that night, every seat in the house was filled, mostly with Latino teens and their dates.

Spanky, the stage manager, greeted me backstage at check-in. "Hey, man, good show this mornin'," he said, clapping me on the back. He held his clipboard to him. "Look, Chief, we need a bio on you, you know, nickname, favorite gym, previous competitions, all the essentials."

In bodybuilding, everyone has a nickname. As Arnold is "The Austrian Oak," Frank Zane is "The Chemist," Rich Gaspari "The Dragonslayer," Mike Christian "The Iron Warrior."

I considered the options. Golem—not bad. Grendel had a certain ring, too.

"Rocky Mountain Way," Vinnie declared, before I could open my mouth. "He's an award-winning powerlifter," he added, "make sure you got that down, right?"

I left Vinnie, my publicist, with Spanky, and trekked off to the pump-up room. On the way, I spotted number 10, my morning rival. He returned my steely gaze with one of his own. His smaller brother, a wispy middleweight in the show, appraised my physique once, then whispered in his ear. Last-minute tips, I suspected.

As the lighter weights left for the stage, I was lost in my own world. If time ticked at all, it ticked outside me. Nothing mattered except getting my pump, feeling the blood course through my veins, growing ever larger before the bathroom mirror. Number 8, the chubster, came up to both number 10 and myself and told us that one of us would win that night. Good luck to you both, he said.

I was pumping up my arms, watching my biceps expand from my arm curls, when I noticed number 10 approaching. He came right up to me, and flexed in the same mirror. What insufferable hubris! I followed him to his towel and towered over him from behind. Then, rather than face him directly, I stood in front of his mirror, all but obliterating his image, and contorted my body into a vicious most-muscular. Point. Counterpoint. If it was war, then war it would be. If it came to blows, I would kill him. I would hang him by the chain dangling from the cistern above the commode.

Before a blow could fall, Spanky came rushing in for our weight class. The night show, nearly completed for the others, had just begun for us. The three of us followed Spanky and his clipboard to the edge of the stage. The rabid crowd, in anticipation of a bloody muscle-fest, had to be stilled by the unflappable voice of Mr. Pearl.

As we walked on stage, shouts of "Oh yes!" and "Sweet!" and "Beef!" filled the air. The three of us "stood relaxed" and beamed for a full two minutes. Then, at the MC's direction, we cleared the stage for number 8 and his posing music. While he performed his counterclockwise turn to "Love TKO" by Teddy Pendergrass, number 10 and I were both hard at work backstage, trying to keep our pumps. He did last minute pull-ups to achieve a V-look to his latissimus dorsi; I did push-up after push-up for my chest. Judging by the silence of the audience, number 8 hadn't impressed. As they say in the gym, "You can't flex flab."

I was next. After all these years, my spot in the sun. I took a few deep breaths just off stage and adjusted my number. Bill Pearl introduced me.

"Ladies and gentlemen," he cried, "hailing from New York City and South Pasadena! A champion powerlifter, a personal trainer at Shangri-La Fitness Training Center. By day, Sam Fussell, by night, 'Rocky Mountain Way'!"

I held my head high once more and resorted to the Arnold Mental Visualization Principle. I actually saw the skulls of my vanquished enemies crushed to dust beneath my feet as I made my muscular way across the stage.

Up on the dais, I drew to one knee, my head tilted down, where I remained, coiled like a sprinter in his starting blocks, for ten motionless seconds. "Giant in Respose." Not a sound from the theater, save for Vinnie's "like the fuckin' orchid!" which he screamed from the wings. So far, all according to plan. I looked once to the side of the stage, signaled the sound man and the music began.

Slowly, I rose and spread the wings of my back into a front-lat spread. "One, two, swivel, three, four, swivel, five," I counted to myself. I hit my arms extended Arnold pose, smiled, then let it flow into a side chest. One, two, swivel, three, four, swivel, five. After my diet, my chest was legitimately 52 inches. No one could touch me there. I turned my back to the audience for the back double-bicep shot and the back-lat spread, twisted into the one arm extended "breadloaf" pose and "Hair." Forty-five of my 90 seconds were gone.

"Shaft!" Isaac Hayes sang on the soundtrack, as I made my final counterclockwise quarter turn, crunched my abs, flexed my legs, and pointed at my calves. As suavely as possible, I cradled my head in my arms, and gave them Steichen's "Garbo." I concluded with "Shake and Bake," a maneuver which started first with the quivering of my legs, then my torso, then my arms, finally leaving my whole body shuddering on stage. But when the music suddenly changed beat, so did I, breaking off the convulsions to stand for four seconds perfectly still, before I crunched myself into a final most-muscular, extending my swollen arms toward the audience in the crab. I left the stage with a smile and heard the crowd roar.

I stood in the wings, sucking in air from the effort, and watched as Bill Pearl introduced my rival, number 10. He called himself "The Black Knight." He had won his weight class at Mr. Midway City the previous year. I was up against a seasoned competitor.

Sure enough, his posing was polished. "Love Theme from *St. Elmo's Fire*" was his selection, and it was clear at once that he had spent some time with a professional choreographer. He had me on this round. I knew it as soon as I saw him glide and heard the audience explode. His posing was so mellifluous, so fluid, that it exposed my rotate and stop, rotate and stop style. But despite my stiff and robotic turn, if I had built up enough of a lead in the morning, I might still win.

At the conclusion of his routine, number 8 and I filed back onstage for the final lineup and awaited the verdict of the judges. But first, Mr. Pearl announced, a pose-down between us all. Right, I thought. Remember the sage words of Macon, of Vinnie. Show your strengths, hide your weaknesses.

"THIS IS BODYBUILDING, SAM, USE YOUR MIND!" Vinnie screamed from the darkness.

Barely had the pounding beat of "Tough Enough" started before "The Black Knight" rushed over to my side and aligned his leg next to mine, thinking I would suffer in comparison. A mistake—if he had selected abs, I would not have gone into a direct comparison with him, conceding him the body part. But legs—that was another story. I smiled, shook my quads cockily, then flexed them with all my might right next to his.

Gamely, number 8 tried to squeeze between us and give his front double-biceps, the only pose he could manage without looking fat, but he knew it was hopeless. He retreated a few feet to the side, and spent the time disconsolately posing by himself. I stayed with my strengths, hitting a variety of side chests and arms, drawing attention to my size, and noticed with relief that "The Black Knight" wasn't hitting any ab shots.

But when he suddenly turned around and began to open up his back, the crowd went with him. To compare my back with his would be pure folly, so I hit "Garbo" again, and then a few crunching crab shots, relying on my greater muscularity to pull me through.

Bill Pearl ordered the music to fade, and, like soldiers at parade rest, we resumed our "standing relaxed" positions in center stage. "The final results are in, ladies and gentlemen, and in third place, number 8!" No surprise there. He stared at the ground beneath his feet as he collected his trophy.

"The Black Knight" and I held hands now, both of us looking heavenward for support.

"And, in second place," Bill Pearl thundered, "The Black Knight!" I heard a scattering of boos. "The Black Knight" accepted his trophy with a wry smile.

I picked up the first place trophy for my weight class, and waved to my crowd. The other competitors filed off, leaving me alone on stage to go through some of my best poses. Giddy from euphoria, I was also gasping, having posed furiously in one round or another for the last 10 minutes. But I would have no rest. At Mr. Pearl's command, the three other weight-class winners (light, medium, and light-heavy) bounded on stage to join me in the final pose-down for the overall, six-foot-high trophy.

At a glance, I took them all in. The light-heavyweight had few muscles, the lightweight none at all. If anyone could challenge me, it was the middleweight, who called himself "Giant Killer," the brother and coconspirator of "The Black Knight." He had a symmetrical frame and good cuts, but I'd seen bigger racing jockeys. The pose-down would be a formality, I was convinced.

As soon as I heard the music, I took charge. I stepped out of the lineup, and placed myself directly in front of "Giant Killer." I flared my lats, and completely blocked him from the audience's view. I wanted him to feel in total eclipse. It was a success. I wiped him out with my size. As he emerged from my shadow, and flexed his leg next to mine, I still had him. Then he hit a series of ab shots, to which I countered with my arms extended pose. I could feel him gaining on the audience. A group began to shout his name. I returned to my bread-and-butter, my most-musculars, but it was too late. The audience had chosen its winner.

I came in second place in the overall contest, losing, like Arnold in the 1968 Universe, to a man 70 pounds lighter than myself. I was Mr. San Gabriel Valley, heavyweight class winner, 1988. But I was not Mr. San Gabriel Valley of 1988. That proud title belonged to "Giant Killer."

13.

THE DIET

WE ACHIEVE OUR DIMENSIONS FOR VERY
SPECIFIC REASONS WE OURSELVES ORDAIN.

—JIM HARRISON

The verdict was in. I was big, all right, but smooth. As smooth as a plate of glass. Back in the locker room of Shangri-La the next morning, I faced the mirror and realized the truth: I was fat. Not U.S. taxpayer fat, around 25 percent, like so many of my clients, but bodybuilding fat. Around 8 percent. It had cost me the overall title at the San Gabriel Valley.

I wasn't really defined, I wasn't really cut, I wasn't really shredded. My abdominal section fairly shouted it. While some bodybuilders have plates of abs between which you could, if so disposed, stick your finger up to the first knuckle, my stomach looked bloated. There were minor ridges, but they were barely visible, and in the comparison round, next to someone like "The Black Knight," who had the real item, my abs looked like they belonged to Friar Tuck.

If I wanted to satisfy the judges at next week's NPC-sponsored Golden Valley, I would have to achieve an entirely different look, for, of the two contests, the Golden Valley was by far the sterner test. The NPC, or National Physique Committee, is the amateur branch of Joe and Ben Weider's IFBB, the major professional league of bodybuilding. NPC bodybuilders are the best amateurs in the world, bar none.

Six days to go, and I needed to lose at least 10 pounds of fat. It would take that much in order to make my waist appear smaller and highlight my abs. My vascularity was not a problem, nor was my thickness, but my muscle separation was.

Moving my eyes down from my abs to my thighs, I realized that I needed to lose some fat there as well. The split that descends down the middle head of the quad was not quite discernible. The sartorius was not visible at all. I was further behind in my preparations than I thought. Vinnie and Nimrod agreed to meet me posthaste for a power conference.

The three of us convened at a table by the front counter of Shangri-La. My friends assured me that all was going according to plan. Sure, I had come in a little overweight for yesterday's show, but I couldn't peak forever, didn't I know? I would peak this coming Saturday, they would see to it. Make no mistake about it, though, the next few days would not be coasting time. It would be "hellweek," as Nimrod put it.

There was nothing to fear. I would be doing what all body-builders do in the week prior to a contest—depleting my system. Nimrod handed me my final meal plan. For the next five days, a thousand calories per day would be a luxury. I had to shut my carb intake down dramatically if I was to appear "shrink-wrapped" and shredded on stage Sunday.

THE FINAL DIET

Menu	Amount	Calories	Protein	Fat	Carbohydrates	Sodium
Breakfast						
Egg whites	2	34	7.2	0	.6	96
First lunch						
Boiled chicken	3.5 ounces	166	31.6	3.4	0	64
Broccoli	1 stalk	47	5.7	.6	8.2	18
Second lunch						
Halibut	3.5 ounces	171	25.2	7.0	0	134
Spinach	½ cup	42	5.4	.5	6.5	91
Dinner						
Halibut	3.5 ounces	171	25.2	7.0	0	134
Totals		631	100.3	18.5	15.3	537

This new diet cut in half the calories I'd taken when preparing for the San Gabriel Valley. My protein intake remained the same, but my carbohydrates were reduced by 90 percent. That eliminated oatmeal for breakfast—not to mention sweet potatoes, pasta, bread, and fruit for lunch and dinner.

"It's a cinch, Sam," Vinnie said. "Remember, this is buildin' we're talkin' about here. The man who wins the contest is the man who is prepared to sacrifice the most." Vinnie leaned back in his chair and smiled. "Just think of Renel," he added.

If this was meant to inspire me, it didn't. Renel Janvier did succeed in winning his light-heavyweight class at the 1988 NPC USA Championships, but the price was severe. In prejudging, thanks to the rigors of his diet, he fainted. Carted off in an ambulance and hooked to an IV through the course of the day at a local hospital, he returned, still sliced and diced, to win his class that night.

But Renel wasn't the only builder skirting that dangerous edge. Death has come to more than one bodybuilder seeking the ultimate "shrink-wrap" diet, and, in 1988, it nearly claimed IFBB pro Albert Beckles. On the European Grand Prix circuit, Beckles ended up convulsing on the floor of a bodybuilding banquet in Munich, Germany. The sauna, the diuretics, the denial of sufficient food and even water—all took their toll. But if I could just make it through the starvation phase, by the end of the week my skin would look like wet gauze wrapped around breathing fiber, raw tissue, and straining muscle.

The same arguments I'd heard before, I heard again. Of course, I would get smaller during the next few days, but if need be, I could always "carb-up" before the show. I wanted to win, didn't I? And even as I was shrinking, I would actually appear to be growing. If things worked according to plan, by Saturday my bigger parts would look even bigger so long as the fat vanished around my waist and my joints. Besides, I'd done it my way before, and I'd lost. This time I vowed to listen.

At least I would only have to worry about working out for the next three days. Lifting weights for the final four days before the contest would be counterproductive. I already had the size. I just needed the cuts, and the only way to get them was by dieting and posing.

So I started my final diet. On Sunday and Monday I ate the new diet, labored strenuously through my workouts, and slept like a baby. But by Tuesday, without adequate fuel, I began to lag. My two egg whites for breakfast were hardly enough. I worked out in the morning listlessly. I was far too hungry to give my exercises their needed concentration, and every time I began to fall into my usual lifting frenzy, I had to stop suddenly to keep from fainting. I was so weak that even when I halved the amount of weight I normally pushed, I barely got through the workout. And this time, it wasn't the saber or my cannonball deltoids I visualized, it was food.

At the conclusion of the session, I could stand it no longer. I gave in to temptation and headed straight for Vern's Bakery, around the corner from Shangri-La. "The Walk" I did was too weak to be its normal invidious self. It was now more of a stagger. The bakery was closed, but that didn't stop me. Looking around to make sure I was unobserved, I inched my way toward the entrance. I bent forward, pressing my nose against the door, and inhaled the aroma from within. My eyes and mouth watering, I remained locked in position, my nose jammed there for minutes, until I saw Vern himself, keys in hand, laboring down the block under a great load of glazed donuts.

By Wednesday, the decrease of carbohydrates left me with so little energy that I stopped training altogether. No longer was the gym the focus of my life. Now it was the sofa. After I rose each morning, I lingered over my abbreviated breakfast, then weaved my way to the sofa, where I spent the remainder of the day, hallucinating and sleeping. Vinnie and Nimrod and Bamm Bamm tried to make me practice my posing, but I was far too weak. Even standing was excruciatingly painful. The soles of my feet, without their padding of fat, couldn't take my body weight.

Once a day, I rested immobile on a stool as Nimrod coated my body with yet another layer of "Pro-Tan" and gave me encouraging words of support.

"You've learned the way, man," he said, on what must have been Wednesday, coating my spinal erectors. My dry mouth opened; I felt the first trickle of tears.

Nimrod put an arm around my shoulder. "Really, man, we're all proud of you."

My mental state was as fragile as my physical condition. I couldn't bear to hear another word. I cried like a baby, clutching Nimrod to my breast, rocking back and forth to assuage the unrelieved pain on the soles of my feet.

Gradually, everything began to break down. I can't say exactly when this started to happen. But it definitely did happen, and it got worse as the week progressed. Wearing countless coatings of my competition color, three layers of clothes, and my arctic parka, I lay exhaustedly on the sofa I had once shared with G-spot. I was freezing all the time. My diet had seen to that. I no longer had enough body fat to protect me from the outside world. It was 70 degrees Fahrenheit outside; to me it felt like 40.

The entries from my journal of that week testify to the severity of my condition. As the days progressed, my handwriting transformed itself from neat, orderly precision to a wild, incomprehensible scrawl.

My sole solace was my inability to think about who and what I was. That kind of speculation required energy and a consistent train of thought, which were far beyond me. I barely remember Lamar and Macon visiting me for their pep talk. Gathering that I was "out of sorts," as Macon put it, they both dropped in to raise my spirits and reaffirm the nobility of my cause.

Macon, adjusting the hood of my parka, said, "I know the contest countdown is tough, but I can't begin to tell you what bodybuilding has done for us, Sam."

I looked at them. Pre-iron, I might have laughed. Now, I was closer to tears.

Macon listed the virtues on the fingers of one hand. "We've got self-respect, pride, the Three D's—"

"And improved elimination, Dad!" Lamar shouted, feeding Cuddles a Chewable.

"No, Lamar, don't!" Macon whispered.

Lamar looked up, uncomprehending.

"Don't feed Cuddles in front of Sam."

In fact my elimination hadn't improved. I hadn't needed to use the toilet in five days. Thanks to my starvation diet, my body was feeding upon itself—which was precisely the plan, so long as it fed upon my fat.

By Thursday, the hallucinations began. Paranoid visions. As I saw myself shrinking, I felt my armor disappear. I felt vulnerable again, as exposed and assailable as I had back in New York. For a threat to my tenuous existence, I didn't have to go farther than the neighboring freeway. My feverish imagination made it seem more than likely that, right there in 1404 Delacey, I might at any moment be crushed by a wayward Mack truck. I could feel the earth below me shake as the speeding vehicle spun wildly out of control in my mind, flattened a hedge at breakneck speed, and ploughed directly into the breakfast nook. I spent my days bracing for the collision.

I tried to escape through sleep, but it offered no release. As soon as my eyes closed, I floundered in the bog of a recurring nightmare. I dreamt that I was at a packed baseball game in an enormous stadium. I left my seat and the roaring crowd to descend into the silent innards of the amphitheater. It was cool there, the concrete as wide as a sea's horizon, and utterly empty. The candy stand had been left unattended. I looked in every direction. No vendor. I reached my trembling, competition-colored hand out before me, clutched a box of Crackerjacks to my beating breast, and ran, frantically seeking cover.

Alone in a remote broom closet, I ripped the top off the box, and emptied the sugary contents in one swoop down my gullet.

Without fail, I awoke at this point, sat up in a panic, and thought, "Oh my God, what have I done? I've ruined my diet!" I'd disappointed Nimrod. I'd disappointed Vinnie. I'd disappointed myself. But it was just a dream. The same, recurring dream, came back again and again to haunt me. The nightmare caused me to rise sluggishly from the sofa, wheeze my way into the kitchen, and seek solace for my parched throat with a few gulps of distilled water.

At the beginning of the week, when I was still strong enough to travel outside of the house, I had gone on exploratory forays into the local market, where, using an empty cart for support, I cruised the aisles, staring at items I could not eat. I held the cart with both hands and pushed forward, stopping every few feet to catch my breath. With my emaciated face and my wavering walk, I looked less like a bodybuilder than a rank-and-file member of the Bataan Death March.

The tuna (sodium content too high), the hypertrophied chicken breasts (not lean enough), even the potatoes (too caloric) were all off-limits now. Instead, I tottered behind my cart as it careened toward racks of cookies, cake, pastries. I loitered around the fudge rack like a toothless pensioner outside an adult bookstore. I never bought any of these items, I just needed to know they were there. Shoppers avoided me as if I carried the plague. Obese mothers scolded their children for staring.

As I watched my skin shrink around my bones and remaining bits of muscle, I tried to countervene this trend of diminishment by asserting myself in some way. In this manner, I could at least prove my validity by reaffirming my own existence.

Facial hair, shotguns, and Big Man clothing became my obsession. I grew a quick Fu Manchu and stroked it continually to remind myself that parts of me, at least, were still growing. Without the armor I had grown accustomed to, it grew increasingly imperative that I buy the Mossburg 12-gauge I had seen advertised the previous weekend. I spent hours on the sofa, my legs covered by a down comforter, a shawl over my shoulders, studying which shells would best be suited for the weapon. *The Shotgunner's Bible* replaced *The Encyclopedia* as my manual of choice. I telephoned Moses, an authority on the subject, and discussed with him the many advantages of weapon ownership.

And when I was too tired to read about weapon specifications, I could still flip through the clothing catalogs for big men. With a red Magic Marker, I circled all the items I yearned to fill once more. Those shirts with 20-inch collars, those pants large enough to accommodate my 29-inch thighs. But I bought nothing. Just as I abstained from Vern's doughnuts and the fudge, the 12-gauge and the clothes served as fodder for my fantasy of buying power, the only power I felt I had left.

As Wednesday ended and Saturday neared, I retreated fully to the bed in my room. I lowered the shades, and locked the door. Closeted in the comfort of darkness, I felt safe. At least here, there were no mirrors. Bad as it had been in the weeks before the last contest, for the Golden Valley it was worse. I had become like a vampire, terrified to look in the mirror for fear there would be nothing there. I hadn't taken a steroid shot or a pill in a week, and though the Anavar and the Deca and the testosterone were still flowing through my body, I *felt* smaller.

So I hid, freezing, covered in layers, playing my posing music over and over again in my mind. I realized that my wooden posing had cost me points with the judges at the San Gabriel Valley. I needed something far more dramatic for a physique my size.

"Posing isn't Sunday mornin', Sam, it's Saturday night," Vinnie had told me with a wave of his wrist strap back at the aerobics studio the previous month.

I finally understood his message, and replaced my 90-second selection of "Theme from *Shaft*" with "Live and Let Die" by Paul McCartney and Wings. The music change necessitated altering my posing routine slightly, but I had to rehearse the whole thing in my mind, since by now I was far too weak to actually practice the moves with my body.

Vinnie and Nimrod visited my room on Friday night, the eve of the contest. I had lost all track of time at this point, minutes blurring into hours, hours into days. At the sound of their knock, I wearily rose to my feet and, almost fainting from the effort, limped to the door. My first human contact in two days.

Unlocking the door seemed like a marathon trial of motor skills. But the presence of these builders resuscitated me, at least for the duration of the visit. With his extensions and his muscular but short physique, Nimrod tumbled through the door looking like an animated troll. He held a tiny piece of black luminous cloth in his stubby fingers.

"Check these out, Rocky Mountain Way! This ain't the fifties no more. You're allowed to show the knees now," he said, waving the trunks in my face.

I extended a weary limb to take them, and, using a straight-backed chair as my walker, retreated to the corner of my bedroom to try them on. The journey almost floored me. I had to pause every few feet to suck in great gasps of air. Constructed from two tiny black patches and a string, the trunks were a decided change from my previous pair. I hoped I had them on the right way. I had followed the normal procedure, keeping the tag, which bore the title of the briefs, the Enforcer, to the rear. Again, with the chair as my walker, I made it out to the center of the living room to essay a few painful, exploratory poses.

As soon as I twisted my body into "The Javelin," I felt my head begin to spin. Trying to maintain consciousness, I focused my eyes on the blue lenses Nimrod had left in the ashtray on the coffee table. I shifted into a transitional pose first, then a full front-lat spread. My body reacted with alacrity. The "Shake and Bake" I did was involuntary. I was on the verge of blacking out, when Vinnie's scream brought me back.

"Holy shit, Big Man! Now you've done it!" Vinnie said, leaping up from the sofa.

I looked back at him in confusion. What was it this time? Had I befouled the competition briefs? Popped the lining of my intestine? No, apparently I had, as Vinnie went on to say, "done the right thing." I had pleased Nimrod too. He pinched the diaphanous layer of skin covering my subscapula, my suprailiac, my upper hamstrings. He could find no fat anywhere.

"Do Gaspari! Sam, do Gaspari!" Nimrod cried, holding one cupped hand to his mouth.

I slowly turned around, gave them a view of my back, then dramatically hiked up the legs of my competition briefs from behind, and flexed my now-exposed ass cheeks.

I heard first Vinnie's whoop behind me, and then Nimrod's. Just like Rich Gaspari, a current contender to the throne of Olympia, I had achieved a low enough fat level to make even my ass cheeks look like a slanted washboard. Line after line of muscle showed through the transparent skin. I hoped to God the needle tracks weren't visible.

"I say it here and I say it now," Vinnie declared, in the "standing relaxed" position himself, "come the Golden Valley, heads are goin' to roll! Shit, you can't be more than 5 percent—maybe even less!"

While Vinnie spun around the room in joy, I dragged myself to the stereo and inserted my posing music cassette. Vinnie and Nimrod sat as one on the sofa. With a motion of his hand, Vinnie bade me go on.

For 90 seconds I endured sheer misery. I forced myself to flex. I whirled and turned, panting and coughing all the while. As Vinnie had taught me, I showed the imaginary judges my Platzean thighs, my Arnold chest, my Joe Bucci biceps. Vinnie was pleased, but Nimrod kept shaking his head through the performance. I realized something was amiss. Nimrod stood up as soon as my music faded and I'd completed the full circle.

"No, Rocky Mountain Way, no!" he shouted, "you're showing the judges all the parts you got to hide!"

Exhausted, I fell to my knees.

"You've got to hide *everything* you got from the judges," Nimrod said, cataloging my flaws, "everything except your bent arm shots, your chest shots, your most-musculars and quads."

As he explained it to me, thanks to my starvation diet of the last week, I had attained fantastic cuts, but I had also lost huge chunks of size. My lats, weak before, were now laughable. Last week, my triceps were hanging sections of beef. Now they were emaciated strands, connecting atrophied tissue from shoulder to elbow. My once-huge neck was now almost skinny enough to accommodate a napkin ring as a choker.

But the muscles that remained, my chest and legs, were shredded beyond compare. When I flexed these, fibers rippled and danced just beneath the skin. The cuts were one knuckle deep. Something had been lost; something had been gained. With no fat, my abdominal section was utterly "sliced." My intercostals alone looked like corrugated cardboard. Nimrod assured me that my new look would not go unnoticed by the judges.

"In the long run, Sam, they are the ones who are goin' to judge you, not the audience. The audience will jus' appreciate your general massivity and overall Big Man demeanor," Vinnie said.

Nimrod gave me a final coating with the sponge-tipped applicator. As I shakily stumbled to the bed, too tired to stand on my aching feet for another second, he promised to bring the boys and pick me up well in time for prejudging the next morning.

"Don't blow it now, Sam. Keep your mitts off the cookies, keep your head intact, and, I kid you not, you'll get your saber come tomorrow eve," Vinnie whispered. He tucked me into bed and he and Nimrod softly made their way out.

I could hardly wait for tomorrow. Not just for the contest but for the toothpaste. I hadn't used my Crest for the last six weeks. It was off-limits. The sodium content was simply too high.

14.

THE GOLDEN VALLEY

I MET A TRAVELLER FROM AN ANTIQUE LAND
WHO SAID: TWO VAST AND TRUNKLESS LEGS
  OF STONE
STAND IN THE DESERT.

  —PERCY BYSSHE SHELLEY

The next morning, I sat at the breakfast nook, brown sweat dripping from my coated brow to the two poached egg whites in my bowl. My metabolism had gone haywire. I couldn't eat even that without breaking into a sweat.

I was too weak to walk at all now, so Vinnie collected my wasted frame in his arms and carried me, bundled in sweat clothes and my woolen shawl, to the car. We both knew that I was on my own once we reached the theater in Burbank. This method of conveyance would not win me points with the judges.

Our caravan circled the theater once before parking. I had graduated. This was a legitimate high school auditorium. Outside, I found about seventy competitors, hovering in single file by a theater wall, all (save for the black contestants) colored various shades of orange. All were "standing relaxed." I had found my own people. They looked like me, they walked like me, they wheezed like me.

Judging by the lean, drawn faces, there would be a number of shredded contestants. Everywhere I could see, skin stretched over ridges of cheekbone and descended precipitously down deep glens where once there had been cheeks. It was not hard to see the skull beneath the skin, but was there anything else left? It would be a giant step up from the San Gabriel Valley if, beneath the mounds of clothing, the contestants had retained some muscle mass.

Vinnie and Nimrod left me in the registration line with my bag containing rice cakes, distilled water, and Gerber baby food—my diet for the day—and headed to the main entrance to pick up their tickets at the front desk. For the 45 minutes I waited outside with the other competitors, not one word was spoken. I felt the stares and I understood. This was war, and each of us considered himself alone in a hostile camp.

One by one, according to weight class, mine last, the competitors filed into the building for the ceremonial registration and weigh-in. After 40 minutes, in which we, as male open heavyweights, sat on our bony haunches, the promoter, a fat gym owner sporting a prodigious belly and a mincing step, finally let my group proceed. There were ten of us in my weight class alone, all of us weighing-in at over 198 pounds.

We silently shuffled into a decrepit hallway that now housed a long table and the Medco weight scale. We filled out our NPC registration forms, received our competition numbers, which we attached to our posing trunks, and delivered the $15 entry fee to one of the registrars seated behind the table. Then, we stood along the wall and closely examined the naked physique of each contestant as he was called to take his place on the Medco.

I saw my competition before me; no one looked invincible. I was sure that I was the most cut, but I couldn't detect much else, not yet. The room was too crowded. I knew I would be the tallest, but that was irrelevant. The best body would win, not the tallest competitor. The San Gabriel Valley had proved that. At the mention of my name by the chief judge, I stripped and mounted the scales. I felt the stares. Two hundred twenty pounds. I had lost twelve pounds in six days.

I retrieved my layers, donned them, and headed off the stage to the seats. The boys and G-spot sat in a muscular cluster three rows back. The lightweight women were already on. Male heavyweights would not be on for two hours. G-spot offered me a rice cake, as Vinnie gave me some last minute advice.

"You're the fucking King of Kings, man. You need a new coat on your chest? Lemme see—no, you're okay there. Oh Jesus, isn't this great!"

Nimrod handed me a vial of pills. "They're niacin, friend. Pop four of them right now and watch your veins explode. Don't worry if you feel a little . . . uh, overheated. That's normal."

I threw five of the little white 250-milligram pills down my throat, chased them with some distilled water, and tried to relax.

Contestant after contestant took to the stage, but I barely noticed a thing. I sat in my chair too preoccupied to watch, too anxious to leave. Within minutes, the niacin kicked in and I was breathing fire. It felt as if I'd swallowed a dozen hot tamales. My body was no longer freezing, just flushed a blotchy red and sweating uncontrollably.

I knew I hadn't practiced my posing enough. Over the last week, my diet had left me so drained that I had failed to go through my routine for more than a few dry runs. There were complete movements that I could no longer perform because of my debilitated physical condition. "Shake and Bake" would have to be eliminated. If I didn't kill it, it would kill me.

When the open male middleweights strode to the center of the stage, the announcement went out for all heavyweights to report back to the pump-up room. This was it. I gave Nimrod a high five, Vinnie a hug, Cuddles a pat. G-spot kissed my sunken cheek, and, gym bag in hand, I was off.

Backstage, in a dressing room filled with mirrors and light bulbs, we stripped down to our posing trunks, and began the pump-up process. Out of the corner of my eye, I spotted a short, thick contestant, number 60, flooding his biceps with quick repetitions. He was big, yes, but flat, at least so far, and 15 pounds off, at least.

I looked at the others in the room. Number 63. Black, five foot eleven, very symmetrical, excellent size. My heart sank. "I can't believe he entered this contest," I thought to myself, knowing that he belonged in a show a notch above this one. I felt cheated, and, in my anger, pumped out set after arm set, grabbing, as we all were doing, any weight that was available. I kept assuring myself that I hadn't come to this contest to lose. Sacrifice, I told myself, was something I knew just a little bit about.

How many of the other contestants, I wondered, had traveled 3,000 miles to become Mr. Golden Valley? How many had quit their jobs? Left their friends back in New York gyms in pursuit of the dream? Endured the grueling workouts I had?

I removed myself from the other competitors to catch my breath back in the men's room. As soon as I opened the door I saw him: a short, stocky competitor bending down, the syringe in his palm, his thumb working the plunger, the needle inserted deep into his calf muscle. It was Escline, the last-minute inflammatory.

"Shit," he groaned, feeling the rush as his calves swelled before my eyes.

He threw the disposable syringe in the waste basket by the sink, smiled at me nervously and headed out the door. A light heavyweight. They were nearly on.

I flexed in the mirror, pumped up now for the first time in days, and as my muscles inflated, I saw that my diet had succeeded—at least from the neck down. I was as cut, as sliced and diced, as any professional bodybuilder. But above the neck, when I managed a smile, I saw a stranger. This blond-haired, orange-skinned face smiling back at me was unrecognizable. The diet had taken its toll. My face was drawn and haggard, my eyes the haunted sockets of a ghoul.

I made my way from the bathroom to the pump-up room to prepare for prejudging. With a smooth coat of sweat covering my body, I reached into my bag and took out my Muscle-Up Professional Posing Oil. I rubbed it onto my legs, my calves, and the rest, hoping I could find someone who would coat my lats. Someone I could trust not to purposely leave great gobs of the white liquid at any unreachable spot.

Except for my main rivals, numbers 61 and 63, the competitors were oiled up. I didn't trust number 63. His easy smile, his huge chest and thighs might well mask the soul of a saboteur. I decided to trust no one, and do the job myself as best I could, when number 61 breathlessly sidled up to me.

"Do your back?" he whispered, sounding like a child molester skirting the edge of a playground.

He stared up into my eyes, and I coughed in reaction to the dose of lavender perfume that adorned his body. He sported a vertical haircut, the curls high on his head, the sides completely shaved well above the ears. His eyes were lost, seeming to see nothing beyond his long black lashes. He was in his own world, now, preparing for the contest. I oiled his back after he oiled mine, our weight class was called, and number 61 dove for the remains of a chocolate bar he had been ravenously chewing moments before. He tore a chunk off, then joined the rest of us in line. He trusted the sudden sugar rush to increase his vascularity. I hoped my niacin pills would do the same for me.

Barefoot, we padded into the backstage darkness together. We paused by the curtain, still unseen by the audience, then, at the MC's introduction, headed out in single file according to our numbers to the middle of the stage. There were ten of us that morning. By nightfall, nine of us would be singularly disappointed.

The audience, about half full for the morning show, applauded loudly for the heavyweights, a weight class that can always be counted on to bring the most muscle to a contest. "Oh yes! Oh yes! Judgment Day!" I heard Vinnie scream rapturously from his seat. The ten of us on stage kept at arm's length from one another and, at the judges' direction, assumed the "standing relaxed" position.

The judges, seven of them in number, made notes as we sweated under the glare of the lights. As a seasoned competitor, I immediately set about projecting the image of confidence, the air of charisma so evident in all true bodybuilding champions. Despite the pain that pierced my thighs, the dull ache numbing my shoulder joints, I smiled and swiveled at selected intervals.

The voice on the humming PA system overhead commanded the five competitors who entered the stage last to retreat to the back of the stage, leaving the first five alone in the center. While I "stood relaxed" with the other four by the giant red curtain in back, the first five were rearranged in order by the judges.

Heartbroken sighs were audible as the judges repositioned the bodybuilders. Competitors and crowd alike knew that if a contestant was placed away from a good bodybuilder and planted next to a bad one, he had already, within the first three minutes of his appearance, lost the show. The judges do not compare good bodybuilders with bad ones. They first sort the wheat from the chaff, then linger over the wheat.

Our five by the curtain definitely represented the stronger group. The crowd had already picked their favorites, centering, as expected, on numbers 61, 63, and myself. As the inferior five went through the mandatory posing round, I stayed tight, still rigidly "standing relaxed." I had to. Even though our group was not under direct scrutiny, one never knew when the judges might be watching.

At the head judge's direction, our group was next. We strode in line to the front of the stage, exchanging positions with the former group. As soon as we stood in the lineup, numbers 61, 63, and I were asked to rearrange ourselves for this comparison round. The excluded two bodybuilders visibly collapsed in spirit as we, the chosen, beamed. I looked to my right and left and saw my two rivals smiling, they knew the effect the Platzean image of American purity and pluck had on the judges. I quickly fixed my own face into a numbing grin and ignored the pain in my muscles and limbs, shuddering slightly from all the flexing.

During the eight mandatory poses, I cockily preened and posed with abandon. It was a relief to actually move my body after the monotonous posture of "standing relaxed." I hit every shot dramatically, as the primitive, bass beat of a jungle drum played in my mind. By the time we filed off to leave the stage for the next round, the 60 seconds of silent posing, I felt the saber was mine.

I was the third-to-last contestant to go through the 60 second silent posing ritual. Pose for pose, I repeated my performance from the week before, but this time it went better. I remembered to keep my legs together. I remembered to move slowly, but dramatically. I hid my weakest points, my back and traps, and accentuated the positive, ending the exhibition with a series of vein-popping, tissue-shredding, most-muscular crabs that rocked the audience. The night show would be interesting. Vinnie caught up with me backstage as I wiped the oil off my body with a towel.

"Oh, Sam," he gurgled. "You looked like a human fucking penis! Veins were poppin' every which way! You gotta love that niacin! You really moved the judges!"

"What about my complexion?" I asked.

"Like a fuckin' tanned newborn," Vinnie replied joyfully.

I noticed in Vinnie's wake a small, mustached man with an expensive collection of cameras dangling from his neck. The little man proffered his hand and regally announced, "I am Tomas. You are the winner, I am certain." I shook his hand and listened as Vinnie told me of all the bodybuilding greats Tomas had shot in Venice.

"I've finally made it," I thought, as I did "the Walk" out into the blinding California sunshine. If only my friends back in New York could see me now: the men by the Universal, Austin, The Portuguese Rambo, Sweepea. How proud they would be! Nimrod and Vinnie stood behind Tomas as I ran through my poses for his camera.

Tomas left me with his card and a wink. He strongly urged that I give him a call the next month for calendar work. He had a project in mind for me that might, in fact, take the whole weekend. He was willing to offer me $1,000, maybe more. . . .

But the contest was far from over, and back at Shangri-La that afternoon, Nimrod ran over my role in the night show. I listened to his words as best I could, and tried to get down a rice cake and an apple. My stomach had shrunk to such an extent, I didn't think it could accommodate both.

"Remember," Nimrod said, "forget the back. And, man, you forgot to do 'Hair' in prejudging. Do 'Hair' tonight, lots of leg shots too. And ab shots, your intercostals really came out this morning. Obliques too, and, man, you'll look even better tonight, you'll see. You've got number 61 and number 63 beat on cuts, not on size, so stay tight and show your torso, not your arms."

Nimrod was right. I had lost the audience in the silent posing round that morning as soon as I hit a front double-biceps pose. My body was too long for this kind of exposition. I had to keep my arms close to my side and flexed to make them appear larger than breadsticks. Any pose that drew attention to my back had to be expunged from my repertoire.

But I didn't spend that afternoon posing. I spent it as I had spent the week before, hallucinating rolling green fields covered in gigantic trees of broccoli, glistening in butter.

We left that night at seven. Check-in was at eight, but as a heavyweight, I probably wouldn't go on before ten. I checked my haircut one last time, spreading the mousse on the top, tilted layer. With the support of my friends, I walked gingerly to the car. We held our heads high on the way to Burbank, driving in the slow procession of winners. Vinnie, Bamm Bamm, G-spot, Nimrod, and I up front, Macon, Lamar, and Cuddles bringing up the rear. Behind us were friends and allies from Uptown Gym, from Bulldog, from Fanatics, from Gold's.

The auditorium, quiet that morning, was a madhouse. Three klieg lights revolved on a circular base by the steps leading to the entrance. Strong beams of white light rose a thousand feet upward. The spotlights were spectacularly dramatic, as the milling audience hoped the show would be. Most of the men were dressed to the nines, with silk tank tops and elevated shoes. Some wore jackets that listed their name, gym affiliation, and personal best on the bench press in script. Their dates wore patent-leather halters or tube tops with hair spritzed and teased to the rafters.

In the packed theater, we found seats in the back. Nimrod, Bamm Bamm, Vinnie, and I sat down, saving a place for G-spot, whom we had lost in the teeming throng. With the hood of my terry cloth jumper drawn over my face, I listened to my posing music on Vinnie's Walkman and went through my routine again and again in my mind. What came after the side triceps shot? Was it down to one knee with back double-biceps, or was it a quarter turn to show back and flexed calves? I only hoped to God I didn't forget any part of the posing sequence, because I'd memorized the whole thing sequentially. Like the alphabet, I knew what came next by what came just before. If I skipped a letter or a pose, I was lost.

The theater had changed since the morning. The official black and gold NPC logo now hung above the posing dias. A red, carpeted platform dominated center stage. And there, stage left, gleamed the gold trophies on a wooden table, the silver saber among them. But I wasn't the only one who'd spotted the spoils.

From behind me, I heard the voice of Macon: "Look, son, over there. Tell me. What do you see?"

"I see the silver saber, Dad."

"And the rest of the trophies, Lamar? What color are they, son?"

Lamar hesitated for just a moment. "Gold, Dad. The color of kings."

"Yes, son, the color of kings," Macon said, as if in a trance.

The teen lightweights took to the stage as G-spot slumped down beside us, ashen-faced. She had gone to the women's room and seen a particularly muscular blond woman donning a pair of canary-yellow posing trunks. "My God, the sight!" she whimpered, wrapping her arms around me. The blond contestant, she confided, sported a startlingly long appendage which emanated from her shaved vaginal lips. It was a result of her supplementation program. Her rosebud had grown to the size of a California redwood.

G-spot was still shivering as competitor after smiling competitor took to the posing platform and offered the growing audience 90 seconds of a distillation of spirit and hope. There were muscular women, with great, wide shoulders and shocking pink nails. Men with huge chests and no legs, others with arms and nothing else. The audience, led by Vinnie, mercilessly decried the flaws of any found lacking.

"Nice bitch tits!" he screamed at a male middleweight's entrance. "You got a bra for that or what?"

There were competitors who had tanned themselves while wearing, obviously, a larger suit for months before the show. Now with briefer trunks, the embarrassing white territory blanketing their midsection was exposed to all. Some had forgotten to shave, leaving a pad of pubic hair above the waist and crawling down each leg ("nice pubes, number 48!" this provoked from Vinnie). Others had overdone the posing oil and looked basted under the glare of the white lights.

By the time my weight class was called, the audience was getting restless, and Vinnie was just one of many catcalling audience members, delighting in the competitors' flaws after suffering them in good humor for the first hour. They had paid $15.00 a ticket ($20 VIP) and were now determined to get their money's worth.

A forty-five-year-old father of two, who, the MC announced, listed his hobbies as (1) bodybuilding and (2) bodybuilding, came out on stage only to be met with great guffaws and shrieks of laughter. "Sausage man!" Vinnie hooted. The sobriquet stuck, and increasing numbers of the audience joined in the chant: "Sausage man! Sausage man!"

He carried 40 pounds more on his torso than he should have, all precariously balanced on a pair of toothpick legs. But none of this stopped him, as he furrowed his brow, bit the side of his mouth in concentration, and tried to quiet the crowd with his posing

display. Sinatra's "My Way" was not an ideal selection. The derisive
chant became unbearable. He fled from the posing dais, both hands
covering his watering eyes. I was just another obstacle he bumped
into backstage on his mad dash to the men's room.

In the pump-up room, a small circle had formed around one
bodybuilder. He was the Guest Poser of the show, professional
bodybuilder Phil Williams. I joined the crowd and watched as he
did set after endless set of seated calf raises. What was that look on
his face? Once I would have mistaken that thousand yard stare for
ruminative mysticism, now, it seemed more like doleful resignation.

He was playing, and was condemned to play his muscle role
until the kind release of death. In the end, he was a prisoner of
bodybuilding, a victim, an iron casualty of the sorriest kind. He
was better built, certainly, than the rest of the harelips, stutterers,
and braggarts who paraded through the gym by day, but he was
equally doomed. Sudden success in the iron game now necessitated
following it up for the next thirty years with crash diets and iron
comebacks. When he rose from the seated calf machine and quickly
pumped out a series of bicep reps, he took up that dumbbell, as it
were, for life.

The consensus in the pump-up room was that the competition
would fall to number 63 or myself. He had the most size, I the
greatest cuts. One of us would lose, but it was still too early to tell.
We pretended to ignore each other, grabbed the iron at our feet
and set about flooding our muscles with blood. There were only a
few minutes to spare and already, I noticed, our numbers had di-
minished. Two lesser competitors (from the first group of five that
morning) had dropped out since the prejudging, realizing the saber
was beyond their grasp this day.

Following my warm-up routine, I visited the men's room—minutes before we were to go on. As I walked into the room, I heard
a stifled moan and the hasty closing of a stall door. Plainly visible
from beneath the stall divider were two pairs of orange-hued feet
on the tiles, the posing trunks of each bunched around their ankles.
If their feet were any indication, one occupant stood, while the
other, facing him, was seated. I was amazed they had the energy.

"Heavyweight talent, you're on," a voice said by the door, and, in serpentine fashion, we all filed down the dimly lit backstage to the side of the red curtain. A man wearing a headset and a beard dashed from his offstage glass booth to make last-minute checks with us on our music selections.

"Hey you, number 65!" the man called to me. "You want me to start your music as you go on, or when you hit the dais?"

"Five seconds after I hit the dais," I replied. Five seconds was time enough to fall to my knees for the beginning of "Giant in Repose."

He nodded his head frantically. "Right, 65, thanks. Good luck tonight, man, that audience is murder!"

"Not for those of us who actually prepared, who strained and starved for the saber," I said to myself. It was on the index card in my hands; the rest were back in my Gold's Gym bag in the wings.

"Ladies and gentlemen, men's open heavyweight class!" the MC intoned.

The crowd roared; they had been waiting for us for hours. Like suspects in a police lineup, we arranged ourselves in order on stage and faced the screaming multitude. I saw nothing, just the outline of the judges' heads.

"That's right!" someone screamed above the buzz of the audience. The audience had selected their favorites, numbers 61, 63 and myself. This time it was Nimrod who yelled, "Legs!" I bit into the side of my cheek as a reminder to keep my quads tightened. I could lose the show on a mistake like that. Unflexed muscle looks remarkably like fat. One by one, we filed off as the crowd cheered for the competitors they favored.

Shining with sweat and posing oil, we watched offstage as the first of us reemerged at the MC's introduction to perform his posing. Some chose powerful instrumentals. "Theme from *Rocky*" and "*Exodus*" are perennial bodybuilding favorites, but this year's choice was The Black Knight's selection from the previous week: "Love Theme from *St. Elmo's Fire.*" As I watched, I grew increasingly confident that I would win the posing round, if, that is, I could get through it without fainting. No one could match my music for pure drama. They were velvet; I'd be a hand grenade.

The MC introduced me and listed my hobbies as bare-knuckle

prizefighting and needlepoint (I felt the Goliath/David combination would attract the judges' attention). But something was amiss. As soon as I emerged from the wings and brushed that imaginary bead of sweat off my upper chest with one hand, my music started. The man in the glass booth had erred. I had expressly ordered the music to begin only when I reached the platform.

According to bodybuilding convention, I had two choices: (1) To stand petulantly with arms folded on the dais and insist that the music start again, or (2) to press on, regardless. I chose the latter, and abandoned "the Walk" to scuttle to the dais. I bounded up the platform, immediately went into "Giant in Repose" and engaged in speed posing. I had no choice—I had to rush through "Garbo" just to catch up.

"Legs!" I heard Nimrod shout. I flexed my quads just in time to accompany a climactic flourish of the music wailing in the theater. At the most dramatic moments of "Live and Let Die," I spun around and crunched my body into the crablike contortions of the most-muscular pose. Blood coursed through my bulging veins, my muscles ballooned, my body turned purple. I smiled my whitest grin (the Pearl Drops Tooth Polish had been a wise choice backstage). I looked like Quasimodo with gleaming teeth.

I remembered to avoid the front double-bicep. I kept my arms close to my body, trying to make myself look as thick as possible. I glided into the side chest position, languidly brought one arm up to flex my biceps, simultaneously passing the other hand through my hair and smiling. Yes, I did 'Hair.' The audience screamed, and I realized I had them. A few more wrenching most-musculars, my Tom Platz bow, and it was over.

Offstage, the other competitors shook my hand. Most had me the winner. But the contest was not over. Number 63, the shorter, larger black man took the stage. The crowd loved him. He was massive, sporting what must have been a 54-inch chest and 30-inch thighs, and showing them to great advantage. He breakdanced through "Sexual Healing" by Marvin Gaye and received a rousing ovation.

Number 61, whose burgundy trunks I now recognized from the men's room floor, was the final heavyweight to perform his routine.

Despite his last minute coupling in the men's room, he bombed. Just as some people dance with ease and others as if they're stomping a cat, number 61 simply could not pose. He tried to match the lyricism of his music with smooth, flowing poses, but his transition movements made him appear like nothing so much as a hopping praying mantis.

As soon as number 61 finished, all of us filed back on stage and maintained the "standing relaxed" position once more while the judges prepared their results. The MC announced the order of merit, beginning with the least meritorious. Name after name was called, until, as expected, there were only three of us left, numbers 61, 63, and myself.

Before rendering their verdict, the judges wanted a pose-down from the three of us. The pose-down might determine the winner, or, as in the previous week, one of us might be so far ahead, it might not. Only the judges knew.

The audience howled, but not loud enough to drown out Vinnie's words. "Like a fuckin' tornado through a trailer park, Sam!" he screamed. Suddenly, Peter Gabriel's "Sledgehammer" blared from the stereo. My two rivals ran after me as I strode to the forefront of the stage. Their chase was a good sign; they were acknowledging that I was the one to beat.

Each of us matched the other pose for pose, and as the crowd grew louder, we drew up right alongside each other, desperately trying to indicate our opponents' flaws. I flung my arm upwards, just grazing number 63's chin, and flexed my bicep in front of his face. He responded with a muscle salvo of his own, bending forward in the crab and displaying his trapezius muscles. Number 61 squeezed next to me and compared his leg to mine. The audience saw rippling flex, cross-striations, bulging biceps, while we panted and flexed, gasped and smiled.

The judge called an end to the round when it became clear that we were all on the verge of passing out. "The results are in," he said, "and in third place . . . " it was number 61, the praying mantis. With a drooping head, he took his trophy.

"And in second place . . . " I heard my name. I lifted my head to the ceiling, gave the victorious number 63 a bear hug, then delivered a fist salute of ironman solidarity to the crowd. Stiffer than a cigar store Indian, I took my trophy amid a scattering of boos and many cheers. As in every bodybuilding competition, every paying member of the audience had his or her own winner.

All the heavyweights, save for number 63, exited the stage, leaving the arena clear for the winners of each individual weight class. But the quick pose-down that followed was a nonevent; the light-heavyweight winner, the middleweight, and the lightweight were no match for number 63. He hoisted the tin saber above his head, and contorted his body as if he were a black St. George slaying an imaginary dragon beside him. Photographers rushed the stage to get close-ups for the next edition of *Modern Bodybuilding*.

Vinnie and Nimrod greeted me backstage. They weren't sure what to expect—a vicious "roid rage," maybe, or a bitter denunciation of the judges. But I was capable of neither. I simply mustered a weak smile as they clapped me on the back. Number 61, the man with the burgundy trunks and the lavender perfume, sat on the metal stool by the master light control panel. He cupped his chin in his hands, and mumbled again and again to himself, "I must work harder, I must work harder." For once, I wasn't saying it myself. Vinnie went over to him and patted him on the back. "Do the right thing, buddy," he said.

I had to know.

"Vinnie?" I asked, as I wrapped myself up in my Gold's Gym sweats. "Was number 63 really that good?"

Vinnie looked once at Nimrod, before looking back at me.

"Sam, I kid you not, that number 63 is just the kind of guy you'd love to share a foxhole with."

I left the auditorium with Vinnie and Nimrod, and met my fellow gym rats at Round Table Pizza near Shangri-La for a celebratory-consolatory feast. Everyone was there, G-spot, Macon, Lamar, Cuddles, Moses, Nimrod, and Bamm Bamm.

The pizza parlor featured stained glass and tapestries on the wall depicting knights prancing on chargers. The iron wheels serving as chandeliers housed candle-shaped light bulbs. Vinnie opened a menu for me, and I took in the "Specialties of the Castle."

In true bodybuilding tradition, the diet was over. I was now allowed anything I wanted, and as much of it as I could eat. IFBB bodybuilder Gary Leonard holds the unofficial record, putting on 54 pounds in 5 days after his Mr. America victory (23 pounds of that within the first 15 hours).

Vinnie ordered for me "King Arthur's Supreme," a pizza with everything on it. Macon and Lamar settled on "The Camelot Calzone," while the rest of the bunch ate "Guinevere's Garden Delight," the sole vegetarian entry.

There were smiles all around. I had completed the final rite. I had competed. I was a bodybuilder. The only one, in fact, who wasn't smiling, was me.

As I wiped the brown silt of competition color off my face with a napkin bearing the Round Table escutcheon, it was Moses who explained the verdict of the judges. "Sometime, man, it ain't who got the most, but who knows how to show it. You'll see, man, the more you do it. You'll get 'em next time."

But there would be no next time. None of my friends at the table knew it, but it was over for me. There would be no more juice, no more three on, one off, split training sessions, no more competition color or amino chewables. In fact, after all the years, all the workouts, all the pain, and all the posing, there would be no more iron.

15.

THE AFTERMATH

I WOULD GIVE MY LIFE FOR A MAN WHO IS LOOKING FOR THE TRUTH. BUT I WOULD GLADLY KILL A MAN WHO THINKS HE HAS FOUND THE TRUTH.

—LUIS BUÑUEL

I'd succeeded, in a sense. After all, I had become that figure I once drew on the cocktail napkin back in New York in front of Sweepea and Mousie. I'd succeeded in gaining 80 pounds of muscle, in benching four and squatting five, in expanding my frame. In the parlance of the gym, I had swallowed the air hose. I had become a bodybuilder, but not, in fact, a very good one.

In their account of the Golden Valley Physique Classic IX, *Modern Bodybuilding* reported: "The heavyweight division provided the most intense competition of the night. Gordon Kimbrough came out on top. He had ample mass and thickness. He was slightly smoother than second place finisher Sam Fussel [*sic*], but had superior overall development. Fussel was probably the hardest competitor in the contest with incredible serrati (pardon my Latin) and intercostals."

Why did I lose? Not because, as Moses charitably suggested, I didn't really know how to show my wares, but because my body (come competition time) was like Bamm Bamm's car. It too was a chop-shop special. A fender from a Plymouth, a trunk from a Chevy, it looked like someone had assembled me much too fast without adequate instructions or understanding (which was precisely the case). My impressive thighs merely brought attention to my paltry calves, my ice cube tray abs to my misshapen chest.

Even after four years, I was raw and unfinished. It would take a good four more to achieve the kind of symmetry and sheen displayed by the professionals of the IFBB. Four more years of eating and supplementing and injecting and playing "catch-up" with those lagging body parts. But I couldn't so much as swallow another Chewable, much less lift another weight. I knew it that night at Round

Table Pizza, and I knew it the next day at Shangri-La when I resumed training my charges.

"Is *this* good for you?" Moët asked, referring to the variant style of pull-ups she was just then doing.

Forgetting for a moment who and where I was, I cast my eyes downward and muttered cryptically, "Is *any* of this good for you?"

What I saw was the older lifters: the builders in their forties and fifties, long in tooth and sparse of hair. They were me in twenty years.

Like them, I could keep on lifting. They spent feverish weeks pursuing size and shape, and then, succumbing to boredom, took months off between workouts. They relied on the principle of "muscle memory" to carry them through their training. (If you read for 10 years, and then stop reading altogether for 10 more, when you finally pick up a book, you'll read much better than a man who has never read before at all. The same principle applies with muscles.) Each and every iron veteran was engaged in a mythical comeback.

Like them, I could keep on eating. As the years pass and the metabolism slows, older lifters get larger and larger, but less and less muscular. The concept of being "big" is hard to shake, so even bulk comprised of mostly fat is preferable to being a pencil-neck.

And, like them, I could die prematurely. Heart attacks, strokes, liver and kidney problems, the ways are many. Eugene Sandow himself, back at the turn of the century, was said to have died of a brain aneurysm he incurred in single-handedly pulling his car out of a ditch.

"It's a quality-of-life issue," Vinnie once told me. "You might be king for just a day, but, by God, you're a fuckin' king."

Once it had all been one to me, just point me in the direction of the gym and I had reason to breathe. But no longer. Now I wanted to feel and care. Now being alive made more sense to me than iron, and I wanted to be alive.

I wanted to eat a meal for the simple pleasure of savoring the food, rather than worrying about its net protein utilization value. It wasn't just doughnuts and chocolate eclairs. It was Brie cheese and wine, ham and French bread. I longed for salt and butter, those staples that actually give food taste.

After all the histrionics and the grandstanding, I longed for a life unrehearsed. I could no longer reduce life to 90 seconds, to ten different poses based on a track of 360 degrees—not with a good conscience. No more than I could abbreviate and trivialize life to a series of sets and numbers, index cards and mottos. Everything I'd done for the last four years had been an effort to keep the world at bay, to find a place in which I wouldn't have to react or think or feel. But having done that, having come 3,000 miles, having gained 80 pounds, I wanted out. I wanted out of that body, that mind, that regimentation. Because as big as I'd gotten and as impressive and imposing as I looked "standing relaxed," I felt that if you could somehow find a chink in my armor and pry apart a muscular pauldron from a gorget, you'd find nothing within that vast white empty space but a tiny soul about the size of an acorn.

It took the Golden Valley to bring me back to reality. The "thousand yard stare" I'd seen on the face of professional bodybuilder Phil Williams, the one I'd seen in the eyes of so many of my fellow iron casualties, I saw in my own eyes in the mirror the day of the show. We all looked like men who'd spent too much time in the trenches.

"TIGHT! STAY TIGHT!" builders scream at one another as they perform their exercises. It's a plea for good form. Close, tight form prevents injuries; it ensures the feeling of security a lifter craves. But "staying tight" also demands a singleness of purpose that obliterates everything but "the way." Save for debate about reps, sets, protein utilization and glycogen retention, alternative opinions are not to be found in the lifting world. Among addicts, the only interest is the next fix.

I should have known better, of course. I should have known better than to think that getting bigger and bigger was the answer to my problems. Sure, my size had succeeded in silencing Jerry, but it hadn't cut me off from everyone. Two years earlier, back in New York, I was on my way to the gym. Thermos and gym bag in hand, I cleared my mind of everything but the upcoming leg routine. But rounding a corner to the Y, I saw an older man, wearing a Brooks Brothers suit, pushed to the ground. He landed hard on his side in the gutter. It knocked the wind out of him. His assailant, twenty years younger and similarly dressed, scooted away. The victim, his nose bloody, clutched my pants leg. Once his rasping struggle for breath faded, he used my arm to clamber back on his feet, inadvertently shattering my thermos on the cement sidewalk in the process.

"Hit him!" the old man howled, pointing in the direction of the younger man. "It's my son, the bastard. Hit him, mister," he implored, "hit him now!"

It was too late. The son sped round the corner. "Fuck you, scum!" his father screamed in his direction, wiping his nose.

He looked at me as if I were at fault, and then suddenly set out after him. "You were a mistake!" I heard him cry when he rounded the corner.

I felt sick to my stomach. It wasn't the thermos, lying at my feet in pieces. It was me. I needed more insulation, more muscles. I would just have to get that much bigger. I rushed off to the gym more intent than ever to find some protection.

But this shell that I created wasn't meant just to keep people at bay. After all, a can of Mace could do that. No, this carapace was laboriously constructed to keep things inside too. The physical palisades and escarpments of my own body served as a rocky boundary that permitted no passage, no hint of a deeper self—a self I couldn't bear. It wasn't that I was worse than other people. It was that I was just as bad, just as frightened, just as mean, just as angry, and I hated myself for it. Every sin that had a name, I saw in me.

But self-hatred is its own form of egotism. As long as I hated myself, I still believed that I mattered. My deepest fear was that I didn't matter. All my life, I'd felt like I was treading water in a bottomless sea. I'd spent my days and nights flailing my limbs in terror just to keep my chin above water. With the sky stretching forever above me, and the water below me yawning to a fathomless deep, I needed whatever buoy or marker or myth I could find to keep me from feeling meaningless in the face of infinity.

I called myself a realist. I reasoned that if, living the life of a bodybuilder, I was a monster of selfishness, I didn't really differ so substantially from my friends who spent their days buying and selling used coins and soybeans and their nights bragging about it in bars.

My posing and preening, my bluster and boasting seemed relatively honest, all things considered. But I was actually much more like them than I was willing to admit. Their money was my muscles. Both of us were stocking and hoarding our respective units of worth, and trumpeting ourselves for our skill in attaining it. We couldn't live without the idea of a credit rating.

I was actually an impossible idealist, who turned to bodybuilding as a way of purifying myself. Like The Counter back at the Y, I was Lady Macbeth in a lifting belt, forever trying to wash out my spot. And if I couldn't eradicate my sins, then perhaps I could conceal them by fabricating an exterior so outlandish that no one would notice what was behind it. But behind that huge frame and those muscular sets, I felt shut up in a kind of claustrophobic panic. Not flexing but drowning. I felt like an actor victimized by his own success, condemned to play a role again and again and again. A role I spent four years seeking out and perfecting, but a role I was no longer willing to play.

I became a bodybuilder as a means of becoming a caricature. The inflated cartoon I became relieved me from the responsibility of being human. But once I'd become that caricature, that inflated cartoon, I longed for something else. As painful and humiliating as it is to be human, being subhuman or superhuman is far worse.

Back in the bunker in New York, my mother had known just this. She recognized in me a certain terror that reduced the rest of the world to a perpetual threat, dismissed and warded off with muscles and mantras. She understood that my monomania was driving me to the point of extinction. She saw that once again I was burrowing myself into a cocoon. Caught up in it myself, I had failed to see the symptoms of my own disease.

I explained to myself and to her that it was in the gym that I was most alive. With 500 pounds on my back in the squat rack, only the moment mattered. But even that exercise was performed in a set-repeated groove, while I employed my belt, wraps, and ammonia for protection.

In the end, I was like those chess players I saw in Washington Square Park. My lifting was life-denying rather than life-affirming. It didn't have to be lifting or muscles, of course. It could have been tax law or eighteenth-century English literature or arbitrage—anything where the obsession precluded all else. I was as twisted, warped, and stilted as a bonsai tree. Another of life's miniatures.

The irony was that I recognized the symptoms of the disease in Lamar and Macon, but not in myself. The one time I'd asked them both about the whereabouts of Lamar's mother, the two eyed each other quickly, then riveted their eyes to the ground, simultaneously reciting: "Fool me once, shame on you. Fool me twice, shame on me." What was interesting to me wasn't the fact that Macon's wife had run off with a vitamin salesman, but that her husband and son were protecting themselves from the possibility of ever being hurt again.

Like them, what I was really afraid of was risk: risking to be myself, risking to say what I actually felt, risking to feel something for someone else, risking to let someone else feel something for me. It was no accident that my love back in New York was someone else's fiancée. It guaranteed a kind of distance on my part. The real connection between lovers was something I could never stomach. The rare times I tried, the pain was awful, the recompense of joy infrequent. Even Vinnie's penchant for pornography was unsettlingly close to my own.

Despite all I knew, leaving iron wasn't that simple, of course. No iron veteran, after all, just walks away. Without the buttresses and corbels, the brackets and bolstering devices of muscles, bodybuilders feel they'd collapse quicker than a house of cards. It's no wonder the rate of recidivism is astronomically high, and all my gym friends assumed I'd be no exception. I was suffering from postcompetition trauma, they said among themselves. Give me a month, maybe three, and I'd be back with my wrist straps and knee wraps once more.

Vinnie did his best to lure me back to the fold. He brought a newspaper to my room signaling the creation of a men's cologne called IRON. It was just then sweeping the country, capitalizing on America's bodybuilding fever. "PUMP IRON," the ads proclaimed. But my eyes skimmed over this to the adjoining article. It was news of Alexei Stakhanov, the Russian hero. According to *Trud*, the labor newspaper, he had died lonely and miserable, a ruined alcoholic. So much for the human dynamo and the sanctity of labor.

Vinnie couldn't persuade me. The months passed, and I didn't return to the gym. In the first two weeks after the contest, I was too busy eating even to consider it. I put on 37 pounds in 14 days. If I was awake, I was eating. Then, suddenly, the novelty of unlicensed gourmandizing wore off. Over the following four months, I stopped eating and lost 50 pounds, much of it muscle. As hard as it had been to pack on, it was that easy to lose. At the end of it, I looked like I'd never lifted a weight in my life. And as odd as it once felt to be a bodybuilder, it now felt odd *not* being one. I moved awkwardly, like a singer who doesn't know what to do with his hands. "The Walk" was an impossibility. There was nothing left to display. I watched the hair grow back on my chest and legs with bemusement.

I wasn't the only one who was confused. A woman who had once greeted my muscle persona at a party with "This isn't a turn-on, you know. I think it's a really desperate maneuver on your part," now reeled back at my pared-down version. "Wow, there's nothing left!" she grieved. "What have you done?" If muscles are property, I'd regressed from a land baron to a serf.

The only ones who felt comfortable about all this were my parents. At the news that I'd abandoned bodybuilding but started a book on the subject, my father sent me a wire celebrating what he called my "iron étude." "All is forgiven," he said, "literature is bigger than people." As an author, I'd resumed my rightful place among the patricians. My mother was simply relieved. She no longer had to roll her eyes when her Princeton friends asked if I were "still tilting at windmills."

And the rest of my friends? Vinnie found Jesus and the "Bodybuilders for Christ Team." He called me once, from Dallas and the mission there. He was ecstatic to report himself, for the first time in ten years, completely clean.

"It's really great," he bubbled over the phone. "We don't do no 'roids or nothin'! We shoot amino acids directly into our system! Have you tried it?"

G-spot won the Junior Nationals and made the cover of *Female Bodybuilding* ("A Bodybuilder's Boudoir: Hot Lingerie Looks").